Smoke-Free in 30 Days

"Dan Seidman has given us a thoughtful ~~~~~~~~~~~ able book. Read it. Recognize you

—Dr.   oyee
                                                                                Mets
and Ass   rsity

"A splendid book regarding the challenge of going smoke-free. . . . [T]his is a valuable guide for everyone. I highly recommend this most informative book."

—Herbert Pardes, M.D., President and CEO of New York–Presbyterian Hospital and New York–Presbyterian Healthcare System

"Although smoking rates are at a modern low, that is no comfort for the 43 million people who still smoke, most of whom would like to quit. In this helpful book Seidman describes the various types of smokers and presents practical ways to help them quit. Give this book to someone you care about who would like to quit but feels he can't. You couldn't give a more important present."

—Steven A. Schroeder, M.D., Distinguished Professor of Health and Health Care, Department of Medicine and Director of the Smoking Cessation Leadership Center at University of California, San Francisco

"The importance of stopping smoking for everyone, particularly those with diabetes, cannot be overstated. Dr. Dan Seidman has led the smoking cessation program at the Naomi Berrie Diabetes Center, and it's terrific that so many more people can now have access to his wonderful program. This book will a make a great deal of difference to so many people."

—Robin Goland, M.D., Co-Director, Naomi Berrie Diabetes Center, Columbia University Medical Center

Smoke-Free in 30 Days provides what is missing from so many books that promise to help you quit smoking: a plan to prevent relapse, which is essential to any program for habit change and is a method supported by NIH's research of successful programs.

—Dr. Neil Fiore, author of *The Now Habit* and
Coping with the Emotional Impact of Cancer

"Alas! How I wish I'd had this book 25 years ago when I nearly went gaga trying to stop smoking. (I finally did.) It is so sensible, so readable. I am sure it will shorten, probably even eliminate, the agony for many people who are struggling right now to quit. Where were you, Dr. Seidman, when I needed you?"

—Harvey Cox, Hollis Research Professor of Divinity
at Harvard and author of *The Future of Faith*

"Dental patients who smoke must be urged to quit. That is much easier said than done, and Dan Seidman's book is an important aid for smokers who make the decision to improve their health."

—Ira Lamster, Dean, Columbia University College of Dental Medicine

"As a cardiologist who specializes in preventive medicine, I find Dr. Seidman's book an invaluable tool in addressing the difficult task of convincing patients to quit smoking....Dr. Seidman recognizes that each patient has their own unique story and reason for smoking, and methods that work for one individual may not work for another. I am certain that by using Dr. Seidman's book, I will be able to add years of quality life to my patients who currently smoke."

—Joseph Porder, M.D., cardiologist, Mt. Sinai Hospital, New York City

THE PAIN-FREE, PERMANENT
WAY TO QUIT.

SMOKE-FREE

IN 30 DAYS

Daniel F. Seidman, Ph.D.

FOREWORD BY MEHMET C. OZ, M.D.

A FIRESIDE BOOK
PUBLISHED BY SIMON & SCHUSTER

NEW YORK   TORONTO   LONDON   SYDNEY

This publication contains the opinions and ideas of its author. It is intended to provide helpful and informative material on the subjects addressed in the publication. It is sold with the understanding that the author and publisher are not engaged in rendering medical, health, or any other kind of personal professional services in the book. The reader should consult his or her medical, health, or other competent professional before adopting any of the suggestions in this book or drawing inferences from it.

The author and publisher specifically disclaim all responsibility for any liability, loss or risk, personal or otherwise, which is incurred as a consequence, directly or indirectly, of the use and application of any of the contents of this book.

Fireside
A Division of Simon & Schuster, Inc.
1230 Avenue of the Americas
New York, NY 10020

Copyright © 2010 by Daniel F. Seidman, Ph.D.

First Fireside trade paperback edition January 2010

FIRESIDE and colophon are registered trademarks
of Simon & Schuster, Inc.

For information about special discounts for bulk purchases,
please contact Simon & Schuster Special Sales at
1-866-506-1949 or business@simonandschuster.com.

The Simon & Schuster Speakers Bureau can bring authors to your
live event. For more information or to book an event contact the
Simon & Schuster Speakers Bureau at 1-866-248-3049 or visit our
website at www.simonspeakers.com.

Designed by Ruth Lee-Mui

Manufactured in the United States of America

10 9 8 7 6 5 4 3 2 1

Library of Congress Cataloging-in-Publication Data
Seidman, Daniel F.
  Smoke-free in 30 days / Daniel F. Seidman ; with a foreword by Mehmet C. Oz.
    p. cm.
  "A Fireside Book."
  Includes index.
  1. Smoking cessation. 2. Nicotine addiction—Treatment. I. Title. II. Title: Smoke free in thirty days.
  RC567.S37 2009
  616.86'5061—dc22   2009023081

ISBN 978-1-4391-0111-7
ISBN 978-1-4391-2355-3 (ebook)

*This book is dedicated to
the memory of Jeff Rosecan, M.D.,
a great friend, mentor, and innovator
in addiction treatment.*

CONTENTS

Part III: Becoming Smoke-Free

Part IV: Your Smoke-Free 30-Day Calendar

"One drink is too many for me and a thousand not enough."

Brendan Behan

FOREWORD

BY MEHMET OZ, M.D., COAUTHOR OF *YOU: THE OWNER'S MANUAL*

When I asked Dr. Seidman to join me on *The Oprah Winfrey Show* in early 2008, the topic of the hour was smoking: why people do it, and how they can stop for good. Dan was an ideal guest because, as the head of the Smoking Cessation Service at Columbia University Medical Center, he impressed me with his experience, knowledge, and wisdom. He has long been our expert doctor to whom we refer patients struggling with smoking addiction. I have seen firsthand the effects of his program—how it helps even the most hardened smokers, people who have tried and failed repeatedly to stop smoking, to kick the habit for good.

On *The Oprah Winfrey Show* that day, every member of the audience (more than 300 people) was a smoker! In addition, we were able to to work more closely before the show with a small group of smokers, all of whom shared their stories and their struggles with smoking addiction. One smoker in particular told a heartbreaking tale: she discussed

the shame she felt about her addiction, and the guilt that
paralyzed her because even the love she felt for her daughter was still not enough to get her to quit. She was horrified
by a video diary she had shot, showing her smoking as she
drove around town with her child beside her in the car. The
most moving testimony was from her daughter, who said her
mom should listen to the doctors telling her to quit and then
summed it all up by saying that her mother's smoking was
"ridiculous."

Since that show aired, a law was passed in the state of
Maine forbidding adults to smoke in a car when kids under
age 16 are present. These kinds of public health initiatives
are wonderful, and they can change the social environment
by sending strong messages about health and behavior.
However, while such laws create a need and a demand for
services to help people stop smoking, they do not automatically translate into a tobacco-free life for the individual
smoker, who is often bewildered by his or her own behavior. Changing the law can spark change, but smokers often
need specific guidance on how best to follow up when they
are motivated to throw away their cigarettes. That's what
you'll find here.

Dr. Seidman's new book guides smokers through a 30-day
program, complete with a day-to-day time line, to help them
through the entire process of quitting—before, during, and
after. The text is full of stories and case examples from his
clinic and practice that help illustrate each recommendation.
The goal of this book is to make quitting smoking—a task
that can be confusing, overwhelming, and at times frustrating—as easy and straightforward as possible. To do this, Dr.
Seidman helps the reader understand that the physical addiction isn't the highest hurdle to overcome. The higher hurdle
for many people trapped in an addiction to smoking is the

loss of emotional confidence they experience. Many truly believe that they need cigarettes to get by in life. Smokers who successfully quit must learn to face life's big and little stressors without smoking. The book takes readers through a clear step-by-step program, helping them rebuild their emotional confidence so they can outsmart the addiction and leave behind the mental compulsion to smoke and the emotional dependence on smoking that the chemical addiction breeds.

There are powerful emotional obstacles that keep smokers stuck in their addiction. A person in the process of quitting will feel some discomfort, but the discomfort is OK. We are not comfortable being uncomfortable, and yet this feeling is part of changing our behavior and getting unstuck. Getting through the discomfort of quitting can help us learn to do better with other necessary discomforts in life as well. We have also learned about the powerful role of the family environment in influencing young people to take up smoking and how other smokers in the family can be powerful triggers of a relapse. This book offers a step-by-step program of guidance for smokers who are convinced that emotional and family stresses prevent them from quitting! If you are a smoker and want family members to better understand the problem you are facing, this book can help. If you are a family member or friend and want to understand how best to help a smoker, this book can help. Because this book is written by someone with deep knowledge and experience in this area, it will ring true to the smoker who is truly looking for a lifeline out of smoking.

Dr. Seidman brings a wealth of 20 years' experience to his approach to helping smokers. The wisdom learned through years of running a successful clinic is now available to you in this book, through a program which has already helped thousands achieve freedom from smoking! Perhaps you could do it alone, but why not make this as painless as possible? Why not make this task of becoming smoke-free as short as possible? Like a guide on a journey, Dr. Seidman has been along the path many times before. He can help you avoid the pitfalls and dead ends that demoralize so many smokers and lead them to go on smoking for many more years and to jeopardize their health. This in fact is the philosophy of the book: to make this journey as easy as possible for smokers and for those family members and friends who care about the smokers and wish them every success in becoming smoke-free. Read on and find a wealth of resources and information inside.

AUTHOR'S NOTE

My earliest memories of my parents all feature smoking: my father with a pipe, cigar, or cigarette sitting on the back patio, or my mother with a cigarette at a family party. Both eventually quit, but not until they were seriously ill and it was too late to save their lives. My father died much too young—at 47—from heart disease, and my mother died from the ravages of lung cancer at 59.

Seeing the harm tobacco did in my family no doubt set the course of my professional career. I became a clinical psychologist and a psychotherapist and then dedicated my professional life for the past two decades to helping smokers quit. My personal history and my work with smokers certainly took the glamour out of smoking for me. Fantasies like sitting in an outdoor café in Paris puffing on a Gauloise, which captivate so many of my patients, are always countered for me by images of smokers gasping for breath in the intensive care unit.

If you are reading this book, you must have your own doubts about the allure of cigarettes. Perhaps you have tried quitting before, or perhaps you are just fed up with living with an addiction.

Addiction is a private agony. Individuals and their families suffer with addiction in silence and in shame, hoping for a spontaneous cure, or a restoration of control. Patients often describe addiction as their personal demon, an alien force calling them away from their better nature. But the battle within can only end as Bill W., the founder of AA, said, in a form of insanity—a turning away from reality—or in recovery, a turning around somewhere in the core of your being. Recovery is not a triumph of willpower but a triumph of self-love, and of love from those around you.

Drug addiction, whether to cocaine, alcohol, heroin, or smoking, is like a one-night stand that promises more than it delivers and then leaves you alone, feeling unloved. It may even land you in the sick ward. The dirty secret of smoking and other addictions is that the feel-good sensations and camaraderie that mark the beginning of so many smoking careers are later replaced by a desensitized brain, and a loss of the initial pleasure. In its later stages, smoking addiction is driven not by enjoyment but by habit, vague fears of change and withdrawal, a wish to restore control over the addiction, and discomfort from withdrawal symptoms. Or it can be driven by a plain lack of knowledge about how to get out of it. When smokers reach this point, they often feel trapped, fear that they can't quit, smoke alone or in secret, and wish they had never started.

Many people quit smoking on their own, with little or no help; other people quit with a great deal of help; and some people say quitting is the hardest thing they have done in their lives. But the fact that quitting isn't easy doesn't mean it is impossible either. Using the program outlined in this book has helped many people discover that quitting is really very doable and not as bad as they feared. It is my fondest hope for you that this book will help you find the easiest possible path to good health and emotional well-being as a nonsmoker.

Please note: Although I do advocate the use of nicotine replacement therapy (NRT), and believe that certain prescription medications can be helpful to some smokers in quitting, I accept no funding from the tobacco or pharmaceutical industries.

Introduction

Why Will It Be Different This Time?

Maybe, like millions of smokers, you have tried to quit and have failed one or more times. Or maybe, like millions more, you want to quit but are afraid it will be too difficult, that you won't be able to handle the stress in your life without cigarettes. As a smoking cessation clinician and researcher, I have run successful programs at Columbia University Medical Center for the past 20 years. Most of my patients walk away smoke-free, and stay smoke-free. They are surprised at how easily they did it, or that they could do it at all! I've helped smokers with medical problems, mood problems, substance-abuse problems, and problems with the everyday stress of living.

I want to share with you the strategies that spelled success for these smokers. As a clinical psychologist, my goal with all my patients is to help them change their thinking about how they approach conflicts and problems. A similar kind of shift in perceptions can help smokers lose interest in smoking.

My 30-day program is based on my clinical practice, and on firsthand research with all kinds of smokers. It takes into account the fact that not all smokers are alike. Unlike other programs, it offers simple, straightforward methods that you can tailor to your specific needs and personality to overcome the particular emotional obstacles you face.

How This Program Differs from Allen Carr's in *The Easy Way to Stop Smoking*

Allen Carr, a reformed smoker, published an influential book in 1985. Carr's book focuses primarily on the false mental beliefs that crop up around and perpetuate addiction. But it is not just false beliefs that create an obstacle to quitting for so many smokers. It is also the smokers' automatic behavior patterns (habits) and their emotional attachment and connection to smoking. Despite this, Carr says: "Do not avoid other smokers" and "Do not change your lifestyle in any way purely because you've stopped smoking" (p. 207).

Often, it is not enough to "give up" a habitual behavior, especially when that behavior involves an emotional attachment (however negative), without finding a new, more rewarding behavior or attachment. In other words, it is important to develop new behavior patterns to replace the old destructive ones. This makes it less likely that you will fall back into smoking. Once the old road (old behavior) is blocked off, with a little effort you can get used to taking a new road (new behavior) until it becomes second nature. However, what you can't do is keep doing the same thing, or walking down the same road, if you want a different and a better outcome!

As explained by Norman Doidge in his book *The Brain That Changes Itself,* there is growing evidence from the field of neuroplasticity that if an established pathway or "mental track," otherwise known as a habit, is blocked and replaced by a new behavior, it is not only the behavior that changes. The brain can also reorganize and rewire itself in as little as "just a few days." But Doidge explains that "quick learning" (daily, weekly) doesn't necessarily become permanent, whereas sustained practice of new behaviors (over six months in some experiments) "solidifies the learning" by building "new connections" in the brain. This understanding fits well with the experiences of many smokers: some report a rapid adjustment to going smoke-free. However, it can take practicing new behaviors and new ways of thinking over time to solidify their gains so they can become truly at home in their new smoke-free lives.

One of the most controversial statements Carr makes in his book concerns the belief that because nicotine is part of the problem, nicotine replacement therapy (NRT) cannot be part of the solution. Carr writes: "All NRT (nicotine replacement therapy) does is prolong the life of the little monster (the physical withdrawal/addiction), which in turn prolongs the life of the big monster (the brainwashing about the need to smoke)" (p. 183).

The *Smoke-Free in 30 Days* program takes a very different position on NRT. Our program is fully compatible with NRT, and we also provide much-needed guidance on how to use it effectively. In my view, misuse and fear of NRT are two of the biggest reasons so many people have not had more success with it.

In short, the *Smoke-Free in 30 Days* program is not just about changing the way you look at the smoking problem, although *honing a positive mental attitude* is indeed a key part of going smoke-free for good. This book focuses as well on *efforts* you can make, *actions* you can take, and *concrete strategies* you can follow, including the effective use of NRT, to make stopping smoking as easy and successful as possible.

Once smokers release themselves from their dependence on smoking, they have to develop the emotional security to handle whatever life throws their way, and the clear understanding that smoking tobacco does nothing to help them cope. Although a small number of smokers may need to stay on NRT for a while after they quit, this is always far better for their physical and emotional health than smoking tobacco.

Some people find NRT objectionable, but again, not all smokers are alike, and many people can benefit from this strategy. As this book will demonstrate, knowing what you as an individual need to do, and how you are going to handle your own personal triggers to smoke, is the key to completely and permanently losing interest in cigarettes. This is especially so for smokers who are not just physically and socially dependent on cigarettes, but emotionally dependent as well.

During the *Smoke-Free in 30 Days* program, you will learn what you need to know to be comfortable without cigarettes. The program will help you: (1) build a commitment to going completely smoke-free; (2) attune both mind and body to being completely smoke-free; and (3) develop a game plan for "quit day." You will also learn how to anticipate and deal with the emotional, situational, or physical problems—also called "smoking triggers"—you face, no matter what kind of smoker you are. This approach isn't based on willpower, motivation, or luck; instead, it involves knowledge, effort, and commitment. Smoking addiction has many ways of holding you in its grip. I will show you how to stay one step ahead of this monster and outsmart it.

The journey to becoming a nonsmoker involves two stages: before quitting and after quitting. If you are like most smokers, you will want to buy extra time before setting aside your cigarettes. With that in mind, I don't suggest that you set a quit day right at the beginning of the book. In fact, I suggest that you continue to smoke as you read through Parts I and II of the book: "Your Smoking Addiction and How to Overcome It" and "Preparing to Quit." By the time you have read these two parts, the fear you might be feeling now as you read these words will leave you, and you will be eager, even excited, about taking the next steps to achieving your goal! My clinic has helped thousands of all kinds of smokers, even the toughest cases, quit for good. The methods we use really work. If you read this book and follow the steps I outline, these methods will work for you, too.

But Isn't It Safe to Smoke Just a Few a Day?

Perhaps you feel that going totally tobacco-free is too difficult and you would like to just cut back. But is this really a healthier way to live? Unfortunately, several recent studies have shown that even just a few cigarettes a day carry a significant risk to health. According to Thomas Glynn, Ph.D., director of Cancer Science and Trends at the American Cancer Society, "despite what we would wish, there is no such thing as a safe level of smoking."

One study by K. Bjartveit and A. Tverdal* followed 43,000 people in Norway for more than 25 years. The results are not encouraging for those who wish to continue to have just a few cigarettes each day. The study concludes: "In both

* See K. Bjartveit and A. Tverdal, *Tobacco Control*, 14 (2005): 315–320.

sexes, smoking 1–4 cigarettes per day was significantly associated with higher risk of dying from ischemic heart disease and from all causes." The authors specifically warn health educators to emphasize more strongly that light smokers also endanger their health.

KEEP IN MIND BEFORE YOU QUIT

Many smokers fail to quit because the fear of quitting prevents them from even getting started. Like people learning to ride a bike, they are focused more on trying not to fall down than on getting up and riding. For most people, once you get past the falling-down stage, your confidence goes way up even if there are a few bumps along the way.

A lot of the failure that smokers experience results from exaggerated, irrational, phobic fear. When they do get around to the quit day, it is literally never as bad as they fear if they prepare, and follow through, based on the principles outlined in this book. We will help you hone your mental attitude through a step-by-step program of proven success.

KEEP IN MIND AFTER YOU QUIT

For some smokers those bumps along the way, or "relapse triggers," are their highest hurdles. When we study smokers who relapse after a period of being smoke-free, two out of three of these relapses involve emotional discomfort and negative emotional experiences. As I will explain in this book, we don't ignore a person's emotional adjustment *after* their quit day, as many programs do; for those who need help after the quit day, this book will offer step-by-step guidance on continuing to live without smoking.

If you are an addicted smoker who is trying to cut down on your smoking in the hope of being a social or recreational smoker, light smoking also may not help. Taking a cigarette, for an addicted smoker, is like throwing a steak to a beast in the brain. The beast gets stronger each time it is fed. The only way out is to starve the beast, to go completely tobacco-free.

Addicted smokers who cut down may be getting less nicotine. However, "light smoking" can actually increase the reward value of each cigarette smoked. Light smokers may think that smoking fewer cigarettes makes them less addicted. In reality, each time they smoke, even if infrequently, the beast will be expecting another cigarette, no matter how long it must wait.

The best plan in the world is of no use if it never gets implemented. Don't think that in order to get started, you need to have everything figured out in advance. Many of the great accomplishments in life (which include going smoke-free!) are not achieved without periods of doubt and even a measure of crisis along the way. Try to start with a spirit of adventure. Remember your reasons for quitting, how you feel stuck as a smoker, and allow yourself to achieve progress over time. Try not to demand perfection or that Rome be built in a day. One day at a time for 30 days will get you where you want to be—smoke-free.

Note: Throughout the book I discuss cases based on people who came to me to help them stop smoking. The names and identities have been changed to protect their privacy, and some are composites of several patients.

Part I

YOUR SMOKING ADDICTION AND HOW TO OVERCOME IT

CHAPTER 1

Why Are You Still Smoking—
Even Though You Want to Quit?

Your smoking probably feels as if it has a life of its own. That is because there is an endless loop that involves three elements: tobacco, your brain, and your social environment. Tobacco changes the brain's chemistry and hijacks the body's own pleasure system, the endorphins, creating dependency on an outside action—in this case, smoking—to alter mood. Smoking also becomes a rote, automated, or what psychologists call "overlearned" behavior. An example of overlearned behavior is walking: for the most part, you never think about it; you just do it. Smokers often behave as if they are on automatic pilot as they fish out a cigarette and light up.

But while tobacco and your brain are developing this unhealthy and codependent relationship, they are being helped by a third and equally powerful partner: your social environment. If you are around smokers, it can be contagious. That's why I strongly recommend that when you go smoke-free you avoid being with smokers. Also, cigarette smoke is a trigger for many smokers, even if they don't realize it. The sense of smell can evoke a primitive response in the brain, so it's important not to underestimate the effects of smelling tobacco smoke in provoking craving.

All three of these factors joined together make for a powerful combination. Another way to think of this is to picture a river that may be fed from many streams: when they combine into a single river, its strong current can sweep you away. The only way to protect yourself is to get to dry land. Even if you think you can just dip a toe back in the water (have "just one" cigarette), you may be surprised by how quickly you can be swept up again in the dangerous current.

Most of the time, people think of addiction as being merely "physical." They recognize that an element of habit is involved. But what is even harder to overcome is the *emotional* aspect of addiction, in particular the emotional belief system and the dependency on smoking that goes with it.

Because many smokers believe they need cigarettes to cope with the wide variety of problems that life presents, they often develop an emotional dependency. They fear they won't be OK without smoking. This is a common complaint among those who have tried to quit but still continue to smoke. Some smokers don't even feel comfortable in their

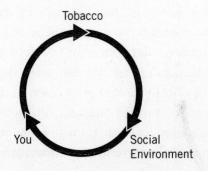

own skin when they stop. This uneasiness can trigger their old fear responses and the belief that they need cigarettes to get along in life. If this applies to you, you will need additional help to make positive emotional adjustments to quitting. You may also benefit from smoking cessation medicine (see Chapters 3 and 4).

Does this kind of upside-down logic sound familiar? You believe you won't be all right without the cigarette, and yet you know the cigarette is a great danger to your health. If this is how you think about cigarettes, you consider them your best friend and worst enemy at the same time.

Your Brain on Cigarettes

In explaining why people smoke, the obvious answer is that smoking feels good. The standard explanation usually goes something like this: smoking a cigarette floods the brain's pleasure centers with dopamine and other neurochemicals associated with big-time addictive substances like heroin or cocaine. As described in *The New York Times* by Dr. David Abrams, an addiction researcher at the National Institutes of Health, "Smoking hijacks the reward systems in the brain that drive you to seek food, water and sex . . . driving you to seek nicotine with the same urgency. Your brain thinks that this has to do with survival of the species."

But what happens over time to this hijacked system? What you don't often hear is that nicotine receptors in the brain are frequently "desensitized." The nicotine receptor, the place nicotine latches onto in the brain (and the place that gives the smoker a "hit"), eventually stops functioning as it does in a normal brain. It loses sensitivity. With smoking, what feels good in the short term often becomes less rewarding in the long term. In assessing smokers who want to quit, I always ask them how much they enjoy their cigarettes. The answers may surprise you. Once they step back and think about it for a moment, most report they still enjoy somewhere between 10 and 20 percent of their cigarettes. This means that 80 to 90 percent of the cigarettes they smoke are often being described as habitual, rote, almost mechanical experiences, which are often repeated without pleasure. In my experience, the loss of enjoyment in cigarettes can become a crucial part of what helps some smokers feel "ready" to quit smoking for good.

What explains this "less bang for the buck," which smokers so often report? Loss of pleasure in the drug experience is commonplace in other drug addictions, such as heroin or cocaine abuse, as well. Smoking addiction, like these other addictions, is greatly influenced by the activation of the reward centers in the brain and also by their progressive deactivation or "desensitization." Picture more nerve receptors sprouting up to make up for the ones on the disabled list. Their job is to cope with the unexpected bath of neurochemicals, in particular dopamine, let loose from smoking. Smoking at first produces an abnormal pleasurable response by overwhelming the pleasure centers of the brain with dopamine, but what happens as time passes? The brain changes, adapts, and becomes "normalized." This means that in order to keep getting the initial pleasurable response, the smoker must smoke more and more—and then, of course, more and more normalization occurs. In summary, over time the brain becomes less sensitive to the experience of smoking, and the smoker often, though not always, experiences less pleasure.

So let's say, for argument's sake, that the hijacking of the brain's pleasure systems takes place at the beginning of a person's smoking career (usually between the ages of 15 and 20). Peer role models and pressure are strong induce-ments to start smoking. It is also well established that chil-dren whose parents smoke are much more likely to smoke themselves than children whose parents abstain.

When they are first getting started, most smokers find lighting up a pleasant social experience. Even if they lose the initial pleasure in smoking early on, however, smoking may still be social or associated with other pleasurable activities, and it still brings at least some pleasure, so it persists.

Most smokers who start in high school think they will quit in their twenties. However, in all my research with smokers, the average age of those who are seeking or "ready" to quit is 40. Why does it take so long to get serious about stop-ping? As important as the loss of enjoyment is as a motive for quitting, ultimately perhaps the more powerful motive is self-preservation. When smokers start to feel physical symp-toms from smoking, or begin to experience feelings of mor-tality and vulnerability related to these symptoms (or from aging), this is generally what jolts them into a more serious commitment to go smoke-free. ,

Premature aging, coughing, and concerns about illness all no doubt detract from the social aspects of smoking. It makes sense, then, that self-preservation would surface more strongly as a motive to quit as smokers move into their for-ties and fifties, which is the typical age range of smokers who participate in clinical research studies.

In my experience, people who no longer get much plea-sure from smoking are ripe for quitting but often still don't know how to get out of their smoking addiction. At this point they are no longer smoking for pleasure, and they experience a rude awakening: they now feel bad from with-drawal if they don't smoke. The system they once hijacked is now fraying like an aging infrastructure. The cells no longer respond with much reward to smoking, but they do respond with discomfort from its absence.

Puffing Away If You Enjoy It or Not

Desensitization to smoking is complicated by the years of behavioral and emotional conditioning associated with puffing away. Each time smokers are exposed to people, places, things, or stressors that remind them of former smoking experiences, these "cues" prompt, independent of the biology of smoking, changes in the behavior of dopamine neurons as well as the urge to smoke again. It seems that even the expectation of an old, familiar pleasure is enough to set off the reward system in the brain! It is not surprising that the classic reason smokers who have quit for a period of time give when they relapse is, "I smoked because I was under stress." This is so ingrained a response that it is fully automated, and stress triggers a return to old, deeply ingrained behaviors.

By age 40 many smokers continue smoking more to fend off discomfort from withdrawal than for pleasure, even if they continue to get only an occasional reward from smoking. For example, many "desensitized" smokers continue to say they enjoy the first smoke of the day because they haven't smoked overnight and the neurons are fresh enough in the morning that they can still enjoy that first hit. Perhaps the biggest behavioral and emotional challenge facing former smokers is learning to find pleasure, and things to look forward to, to restore the functioning of the brain's reward centers, hijacked in their youth by smoking.

There are many people who do continue to enjoy smoking and still confront the need to quit to preserve their health. In some ways their task is more difficult than that of smokers who no longer enjoy smoking but just don't know how to quit. People tend to stick with what is familiar, and that's a big part of what makes changing any behavior, including smoking, so difficult and challenging.

How the Media Created
Our Cultural Beliefs about Smoking

The media, over many decades, have given us powerful images of smoking that have created lasting assumptions about what smoking can do for us. Even though many of the media, because of laws and social pressure, have abandoned their smoking propaganda, the images they cultivated for so long linger in our culture.

From the 1920s until at least the 1990s, the advertising industry and the media conspired to make smoking seem glamorous and fun. Through magazine ads, billboards, and eventually television, smoking was promoted as a way to be more masculine, feminine, sexy, thin, and even healthy! Unbelievably to us today, one print ad actually boasted that "according to a recent nationwide survey More Doctors Smoke Camels Than Any Other Cigarette." This was long before the surgeon general's report of 1964 declaring that smoking was responsible for an epidemic of lung cancer, emphysema, and heart disease. After the report, a health warning was required on all cigarette packages.

Cigarette advertising was banished from TV and radio by Congress in 1971. After a settlement with the tobacco industry in 1999, billboards selling cigarettes were replaced with antismoking messages. And in 2003 the industry agreed to restrict advertising for cigarettes in magazines aimed at young people. Although billboards featuring the likes of Joe

Camel (a favorite of children) and television advertisements are now, thankfully, a thing of the past, cigarettes are still advertised in some magazines to this day.

It is no coincidence that the reasons marketers have given for smoking in their ads over the years are echoed in the reasons addicted smokers give today for their smoking. These ads, spread over many decades, helped make cigarette smoking the most common addiction in history. They created many powerful cultural assumptions and beliefs about smoking. The *Smoke-Free in 30 Days* program is designed to help you disconnect from these assumptions.

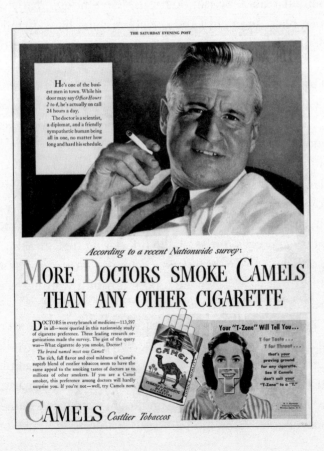

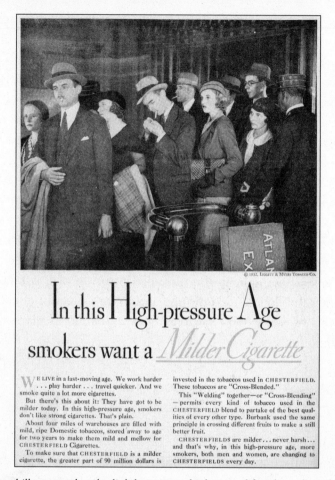

© 1932, LIGGETT & MYERS TOBACCO CO.

In this High-pressure Age
smokers want a *Milder Cigarette*

WE LIVE in a fast-moving age. We work harder . . . play harder . . . travel quicker. And we smoke quite a lot more cigarettes.

But there's this about it: They have got to be milder today. In this high-pressure age, smokers don't like strong cigarettes. That's plain.

About four miles of warehouses are filled with mild, ripe Domestic tobaccos, stored away to age for two years to make them mild and mellow for CHESTERFIELD Cigarettes.

To make sure that CHESTERFIELD is a milder cigarette, the greater part of 90 million dollars is invested in the tobaccos used in CHESTERFIELD. These tobaccos are "Cross-Blended."

This "Welding" together—or "Cross-Blending" —permits every kind of tobacco used in the CHESTERFIELD blend to partake of the best qualities of every other type. Burbank used the same principle in crossing different fruits to make a still better fruit.

CHESTERFIELDS are milder . . . never harsh . . . and that's why, in this high-pressure age, more smokers, both men and women, are changing to CHESTERFIELDS every day.

This ad illustrates that the link between a high-stress lifestyle and smoking has been made for generations.

The role of cigarettes in Hollywood and on television also cannot be underestimated as an influence on a nation's smoking addiction. Such iconic Hollywood stars as Bette Davis and Humphrey Bogart (who died of esophageal cancer at the age of 57) appeared in dozens of films, cigarette in hand. Bogey represented the male ideal for many—dashingly dressed in a trench coat, a cigarette dangling between his lips—while female stars like Bette Davis signaled their sexuality through the way they dragged on a cigarette or blew smoke toward their intended conquest. And on television, even the brilliant journalist Edward R. Murrow (recently portrayed in the film *Good Night, and Good Luck*) appeared on camera wreathed in smoke, a cigarette forever in hand. Like Bogart, he died at 57, in his case of lung cancer, the result of his three-pack-a-day habit.

Although smoking in films these days is mostly limited to foreign imports or historical biopics, a recent popular movie *He's Just Not That into You* came in for condemnation from antismoking groups for its "product placement" of various brands of cigarettes. Even though smoking was presented in a negative light in the film, the inclusion of this kind of almost subliminal advertising can have a powerful effect on young viewers, who see cigarettes as part of a glamorous celluloid lifestyle.

The Role of the Tobacco Industry in Creating a False-Belief Syndrome

Without tobacco, the history of America would have been quite different. When Sir Walter Raleigh introduced smoking to England in the sixteenth century, he created a market that would make the settlers of the Virginia colony and their descendants prosperous farmers for centuries to come. This cash crop would grow into a powerhouse as an economic force in the American economy, representing as much as 2.5 percent of the U.S. gross national product. With its important role in the economy would come political power, memorialized by the sculptured tobacco leaves which adorn the columns in the Senate rotunda in Washington, D.C., which kept tobacco subsidized by American taxpayers. What accounts for the profound success of this product? We've seen how advertisements positioned cigarettes not just as a recreational activity, but as some sort of modern miracle cure-all. This is the origin of the false-belief syndrome around cigarettes created by the tobacco industry using the joint imagination of Madison Avenue and Hollywood. It is this false-belief syndrome that works to perpetuate smoking addiction.

Think about the depth of our mixed beliefs about cigarettes. This all-purpose product:

1. Makes a man more masculine and a woman more feminine. Nice trick!
2. Makes you a rebel as well as a full-fledged adult member of society.
3. Is a reward when you're celebrating, and a comfort in loss or defeat.

Cigarettes have been promoted as a way to relieve stress and boredom, as a friend for the lonely, and as an energy pick-me-up. They are supposed to be as good as sex and chocolate cake, and also make you thin. They give you something to do when you feel emotional pain, and a way to show others that you are hurting, angry, or nervous. This way of signaling emotions was useful in films in telegraphing a character's inner state or motivation. Think about Bette Davis angrily puffing on a cigarette. We knew exactly what she was feeling just by the way she inhaled.

Without the Hollywood fantasies smokers have been sold, how many would willingly ingest a product with a skull and crossbones on it to stay thin or cope with stress? The irony is that thinness from smoking weakens the body from poor health. Using cigarettes for stress management weakens the mind's psychological response to life's problems through rote coping. As smokers get older, many report that they no longer enjoy most of the cigarettes they smoke. A minority of smokers do enjoy the experience all the way. But even those smokers find it difficult to imagine willingly swallowing poison for the experience. Unfortunately, poison is exactly what this fantasy-filled product delivers.

These cultural myths about smoking have worked their way deep into the American psyche, and also into cultures from Beijing to Beirut. And there's more: the marketing machine has smokers convinced that not only is the experience uniquely wonderful, but quitting is impossible (or at least extremely difficult). What if both these premises are untrue, or at least greatly exaggerated? Remember, the smoking rate was cut in half between the release of the surgeon general's report in 1964 and 2004. So obviously it is not impossible to quit, if there are now more ex-smokers than smokers. Now, if you believed it was impossible to quit you might avoid even trying and build up an irrational fear of quitting. It's amazing how many people are afraid to quit but have never tried it even for a day. They may assume that the minor but nagging withdrawal symptoms they come up against each day between cigarettes will become that much more unmanageable without any cigarettes. In fact, they are so afraid to try that they don't even know how they will respond if they quit for real.

Fact: nicotine withdrawal requires no medical supervision, as is sometimes the case with alcohol or drug withdrawal.

The reason: there are no physical risks for smokers who want to quit except the fear that they cannot live without their cigarettes.

Perhaps fear of quitting is the whole story for about half of all smokers. The other half may also have adjustment problems, because they have spent years "coping" with life with a rote habit. When smokers first go cigarette-free, they feel raw because they need some new and healthier (both physically and mentally) responses to life's ups and downs. These ups and downs are part of everyone's life experiences. Learning to manage a tobacco-free life is possible, and this program will tell you how to do it.

CHAPTER 2

What Kind of Smoker Are You?

Knowing what kind of smoker you are will help you plan for success. Although every smoker is of course a unique individual, there are six basic types. You may quickly identify yourself with a particular type of addicted smoker, but reading the stories about the other types of smokers will offer valuable and relevant insights no matter what kind of smoker you are.

The Recreational or Social Smoker

Very few smokers belong in this category, although many wish they did fit here. If you are a social smoker, you smoke when you're at a party, at a bar, or at a friend's house, but you don't light up when you're alone. A friend of mine, a physician, smokes only when he plays poker or goes fishing with his friends or when his two-pack-a-day friend visits. He never thinks of smoking at any other times. He is the envy of all the addicted smokers who wish they could, but can't, be like him. Historically, only one in 10 smokers has been classified as a recreational or social smoker.

More recent health surveys, however, suggest that "intermittent" smokers, those who don't smoke every day, may represent closer to 20 or even 25 percent of smokers in the United States, especially among younger smokers and in areas that have restrictions on public smoking. Dr. Saul Shiffman, a professor at the University of Pittsburgh, has made a special study of this trend among smokers and believes that nondaily use may become a more normal smoking pattern over time in the United States as it is in many countries where daily smoking is not affordable for much of the population.* A key point to be made about nondaily or intermittent smokers is that just because someone does not smoke daily does not mean he or she is a truly recreational or nonaddicted smoker. Some of these nondaily smokers also fit the type, described later in this chapter as "situational" smokers, who can't truly "take it or leave it" (like the recreational smoker), and report a stubborn pattern of addiction and strained efforts to quit that can present a surprising challenge.

Perhaps the most prominent current example of a nondaily smoker is President Barack Obama, whose press secretary explained in the *New York Times* ("Occasional Smoker, 47 Signs Tobacco Bill," June 23, 2009) that "he struggles

---

* In contrast to Dr. Shiffman, Dr. Renee Goodwin at the Columbia University Mailman School of Public Health (*American Journal of Public Health,* August 2009) presents evidence that, while the "overall prevalence of cigarette use declined between 1964 and 2002," among continuing smokers, over these decades, the ratio of heavy and dependent smokers who meet the psychiatric definition for "nicotine dependence" has actually increased (not decreased) and that these smokers have not shown a decline in smoking as we have seen in the general population.

with it every day . . . it's a continuing struggle." This is not a description of recreational or social smoking. Many occasional smokers are a different breed from the take-it-or-leave-it social smoker: they may experience fewer cravings than a heavy daily smoker, but still more cravings than the social smoker who experiences none at all! Some occasional smokers may train themselves "to wait to smoke" through will power and self-discipline, and *never really accept the notion that they must quit altogether.* Instead, they continue to struggle every day with it.

One thing to beware of if you smoke recreationally is that addiction can sneak up on you over time, and before you know it you will have graduated to being an addicted smoker. It is fashionable now to say, "I smoke only when I have a drink with a friend or at a party." Read through the following categories of smokers to help assess if you have, perhaps unbeknownst to yourself, crossed the line from recreational to addicted smoking. One clue will be: have you started smoking alone or in secret, or are you pretending to yourself and others that you only smoke socially?

The Scared-to-Quit Smoker

Thomas M., a charming and gregarious journalist in his forties, always said he would quit tomorrow. He had smoked the same brand of unfiltered cigarettes as his father for 20 years. But he had developed circulatory problems and was facing surgery, and it seemed he was now just as afraid to smoke as he was to quit.

He admitted he would use any excuse, even being ill, as a reason to continue smoking. When he was feeling good he told himself, "This can't hurt me." He wanted to prove he could "take only one." But when he finished that one, he started to feel empty inside, and 20 minutes later he wanted another. In the past he had even exaggerated his cravings, and lack of progress, as an excuse to embrace defeat and justify going back to smoking after quitting. He admitted, "My confidence is shot." In an irrational way he felt that quitting smoking was a "terrible defeat" and a betrayal of his "badge of honor" and "identity" as a smoker.

Even though this kind of logic makes no sense to a non-smoker, or even to someone who quit a long time ago, I suspect that you might identify with some of these upside-down thoughts. Addiction has a way of distorting our thoughts. Let's call it "creative rationalization." Smoking can rival its more acknowledged fellow major addictions—like alcoholism, cocaine abuse, or heroin addiction—in this regard.

Thomas could come up with all kinds of creative rationalizations for smoking on the one hand, but on the other hand he also felt like a "humiliated slave" to his addiction, and so his mind raged back and forth in a kind of civil war. Trying to quit, and asking for outside help to do it, meant waving the white flag on the battlefield, giving up the wish to control his addiction. He realized he had to get honest with himself. When he finally did quit, he said it was honesty, an unflinching willingness to pick apart his numerous excuses to smoke, that made it possible to stay completely smoke-free.

The Emotion-Triggered Smoker

Charles M. sought help because he had life-threatening medical problems, and had relapsed after not smoking for two months. He told me about a frustrating experience he had when his car was towed. He became so angry, he said, "I wanted to tear someone's heart out." He made himself calm down, and he said, "To reward myself I smoked later that day." He looked on smoking as a reward for his good behavior in getting through a stressful situation. But he also knew that smoking ultimately threatened his life. The good news is that he did manage to quit smoking by using a nicotine inhaler that he gradually tapered off over several months.

Smokers with mood problems and emotional distress in addition to smoking addiction have been the focus of our clinic at Columbia, and in my practice. Mood problems can magnify nicotine withdrawal and complicate the emotional adjustment after quitting. Even for these hard-core smokers, each and every one has the potential to be successful in becoming tobacco-free with the approach outlined in this book, and the necessary effort on his or her part.

If you fall into this category, you smoke to avoid conflict and negative emotions. For you, smoking is a form of social and emotional withdrawal. Your biggest challenge is to get comfortable in your own skin without smoking. It is probably difficult for you to picture a time when being smoke-free will feel "normal." That's because smoking weakens your capacity to experience emotions; you rely on it to cope with, and cover over, negative feelings.

Barbara S. described how emotional pain or distress triggered automatic thoughts of smoking. When she first came to see me, her brother had been diagnosed with lung cancer from smoking, and her granddaughter, whom she helped raise, was having serious behavioral problems. Her strong cravings to smoke were triggered by her distress about these people who were so close to her. She didn't believe she could handle powerful feelings without a cigarette to "calm down."

As we worked together to face these crises without smoking, she actually began to feel less stressed and depressed, more able to tolerate "negative" feelings, and more able to make constructive decisions about how she wanted to live her life. Over time, as we talked through how unproductive smoking was for her, she reported more frequent good moods, and that she was not even thinking about smoking anymore.

> *Christine L. was a gifted artist, married to a college professor. When she was 12, her mother died. Like many who suffer a trauma at an early age, she became an addicted smoker, and went through three packs a day. She came to me because she had developed a heart condition that caused her great anxiety. During our talks she would say, "I was born to smoke." Smoking was wrapped up in her sense of herself, her "identity." It was her distraction and her reward: her drug of choice.*

She told me right at the outset, "Anger is my issue even with cigarettes." She would quit, but then the anger would start to build up inside her along with the tension to smoke again. She repeated this pattern several times before I was able to teach her to disconnect her smoking addiction from her anger. How did she do this? By making a conscious effort. She would repeat to herself, "Smoking never helped me solve a real-life problem."

Once she cut off the habitual response, she began to discover more satisfying and empowering ways to cope when she became angry. For example, with her husband or a coworker, instead of taking the bait the same way each time, like stubbing her toe in the same place, she refused to play the victim anymore and to smoke as a booby prize. Pretty soon she started to enjoy her new ability to choose a response and not passively fall into the same old trap. This is what helped her say good-bye to her smoking addiction for good. Once she no longer felt powerless and helpless when angry, she lost her interest in smoking completely.

For emotionally dependent smokers, the solution is to develop emotional confidence, so they can disconnect the automatic smoking response from the trigger of emotional discomfort. Developing one's emotional capacity is like exercising a muscle: the more you use it, the stronger it becomes.

SMOKING AND DEPRESSION

I am not convinced of the antidepressant properties of smoking, and believe they are often overstated. More likely, smoking feeds on smokers' mood problems, and is in fact a "negative reinforcer." Negative reinforcement *strengthens* a behavior because it stops a "negative" condition. For example, it feels good to come in out of the cold and sit by a fire. Getting rid of the negative condition (being cold) makes it more likely you will repeat the rewarding behavior (sitting by the fire). What makes cigarettes a great negative reinforcer?

Withdrawal from cigarettes creates mood problems. Smoking cigarettes relieves and perpetuates these bad moods. Some version of the withdrawal-relief cycle goes on even when the smoker isn't trying to quit. First, waiting for the next cigarette creates a bad mood (you are out in the cold) and smoking presents itself as the answer (come in and sit by the fire). Smoking thus is really a mood manipulator more than a good mood support or antidepressant.

This phenomenon becomes even more complicated in people who already have problems with mood, such as depression, anxiety, or anger, which are independent of smoking addiction. Withdrawal in these people magnifies their preexisting symptoms, and they are then especially prone to believe they cannot handle their emotions without smoking.

Even for those smokers who don't have a clinical mood disorder, over time smoking becomes the default coping mechanism for "stress" and everyday life problems. Most smokers say this as if they are reading from the same script. For most emotionally dependent smokers, smoking becomes a conditioned way of coping emotionally.

If smoking were truly such a great antidepressant, why do so many smokers say they feel better after a period of time away from it? They expect to feel worse but they actually feel better without smoking, once they overcome the withdrawal. If you have a tendency to get clinically depressed, make sure you get the proper help you need, whether it is psychotherapy, medication, or both. Depression is a very treatable disease. (See the Depression Self-Assessment and the Anxiety Self-Assessment in Chapter 4.)

If you suffer from the everyday blues, which are not as severe as clinical depression, the *Smoke-Free in 30 Days* program can help you work on developing your emotional confidence so you can disconnect the automated smoking response from the trigger of emotional discomfort. When you have a loss or a setback in life, it is important to learn to let yourself feel bad, at least initially, rather than "doing something," like smoking a cigarette. By now you know that smoking cigarettes won't cure your troubles, which will still be waiting for you when you finish that cigarette.

The Worried-about-Weight Smoker

Julia D., model-thin and attractive, was about to turn 40 and was starting to confront her own mortality. Her smoking made her fearful about what might happen to her family if she got sick. Her husband had recently been diagnosed with a serious illness, and several of her friends were also having medical problems. She smoked about 10 cigarettes a day, but not at home or in front of the kids. She was a "secret smoker" who hid her addiction from both friends and family. Although she worked out every day, the last time she quit she had gained 6 pounds in 2 weeks, and this, as she said, "put me in a bad mood." She described herself as a "very anxious person" and a "perfectionist and a hypochondriac, so smoking doesn't work for me." Nonetheless she was worried about those 6 pounds.

Smokers who are fearful of gaining weight use cigarettes to suppress their appetite. They are afraid to quit because they will gain weight. When they are younger they tell themselves, "Even if smoking is bad for me, at least being thinner is healthy." This myth begins to lose credibility as these smokers age and see what is happening to their peer group. In fact, thinness from smoking is associated with poor health. Unfortunately, the metabolic increases from smoking are due not to a healthy but to an unhealthy process: the body's need to get rid of the poisons from the cigarettes as fast as possible.

I set up a treatment plan for Julia using nicotine replacement therapy (NRT; see Chapter 3). We also reviewed drinking water as a new ritual; using deep-slow breathing, to calm her stress and worry; and how to avoid other smokers. We set a specific date for her to quit. She succeeded and said the first three days were "not hard," thanks to NRT. She saw that her husband was denying his serious health problems, and she didn't want to do the same with her smoking addiction. She kept her weight down with nicotine gum and saw some weight gain as a reasonable compromise to protect her family.

Some compelling health and beauty reasons to give up smoking:

- Good skin
- Being more athletic
- Good oral hygiene, including keeping your teeth
- Fresh breath, clothes, and home
- More calcium for your bones as you age

A NOTE ON WEIGHT GAIN AND AGING:

There is a normal weight gain with aging until around the age of fifty-five. Women, in particular, also tend to put on more weight than their male counterparts.* As described by Dr. Robert Klesges and Margaret DeBon in their book *How Women Can Finally Stop Smoking*, this "natural" weight gain is typically about one pound every 3 to 4 years. This adds up to about 8 pounds on average for someone smoking 20 years. It is this missing 8 pounds for women (6 pounds for men) that return when a smoker goes smoke-free.

Most studies[†] report that heavy smokers are more at risk for weight gain than moderate or light smokers. Turning to sugar in all its forms to cope with cravings is also a factor in weight gain when going smoke-free. Exercise is the healthy alternative because, like smoking, it also increases the metabolic rate, but without the damage done by the poisons in the cigarettes.

The Alcoholic Smoker

William G. grew up in England and came to the United States as a young man. He married, began a family, and started a business. Each evening after work, he would stop into a bar on the way home and have several drinks and smoke. He also

---

* David F. Williamson, "Descriptive Epidemiology of Body Weight and Weight Change in U.S. Adults, *Annals of Internal Medicine,* 119, 7 (October 1993), Part 2: 646–649.

† Robert C. Klesges, Andrew W. Meyers, Lisa M. Klesges, Marie E. LaVasque, "Smoking, Body Weight, and Their Effects on Smoking Behavior: A Comprehensive Review of the Literature," *Psychological Bulletin,* 106, 2 (September 1989): 204–230.

drank in secret at home. When I met him, he was, as they say
in Alcoholics Anonymous, "sick and tired of being sick and
tired." He was referred to me by his physician, because of his
fears about becoming sober. He said he felt he was "stepping
into a void with sobriety." He knew he was cheating his busi-
ness partners and his family with his compulsive drinking,
but despite his wish to stop, "It just never happens." Shortly
before coming to see me he had stopped drinking under his
physician's guidance, using Antabuse, a medication that
causes you to feel violently ill if you drink. He then began the
long road to overcoming his sense of lost opportunity, guilt,
and feelings of inadequacy from his hard-drinking years.

Two months into sobriety he decided to quit smoking. In
his mind, smoking was connected with his dependency on
alcohol, and his use of smoking as a "reward" bothered him.
He quit as planned and reported after 8 days of not smoking that he needed to have "patience" with himself. After
2 weeks smoke-free, he could feel himself making progress
with his work, marriage, children, and exercise. He began
confronting "something missing" inside him, a "hole" that he
was now filling as his life was improving. Unfortunately, the
first attempt to quit didn't work.

After several promising but false starts, about 15 months
after becoming sober William quit smoking for good. His
burden of shame and guilt was lessening. Gradually his
tendency to worry was transformed from catastrophic fears
of failure and loss to recognizing and coping with everyday
real-world problems as they arose. At 2 years sober, he had
been smoke-free for 9 months.

In the next year he reported a loosening of his rigid perfectionist demands on himself, and more stable moods and
confidence in handling his life. He was enjoying his home

life and work life more, and felt he was making good progress. Although he still had stressful times, he no longer was thinking of alcohol or smoking as a way to handle them. Ten years after his first visit, he continued to be smoke-free and sober.

This case is a good example of the way the addictive use of chemicals like alcohol and tobacco weakens the addict's capacity to handle normal life stresses and anxiety, and how that capacity must be rebuilt over time once the drug use stops. Alcohol often serves to prime the pump for smoking, so even if you are not an alcoholic it can be crucial to consider how you are going to handle drinking while quitting smoking.

But how does a smoker know if drinking alcohol is a problem in its own right, and not just a cue that tells the brain it's time to smoke a cigarette? See the alcohol health checkup in Chapter 4 to find out whether you meet the criteria for alcohol abuse. If so, this may complicate your efforts to quit smoking, and it is a good time to discuss this honestly with a trusted health professional.

Research suggests that recovering alcoholics are often heavier smokers than nonalcoholics. Nonetheless they have similar rates of short-term success with quitting smoking. Research also suggests that stopping smoking doesn't disrupt recovery from alcohol or other drugs, and may even enhance it! At least one study suggests, however, that it may be best to quit drinking first, and to quit smoking once you are sober.

This approach of tackling one problem at a time is similar to the standard advice, also backed up by research, to stop smoking first and address weight concerns later. The principle is to build on success without overwhelming the person by trying to do too much all at once.

ALCOHOLISM AND SMOKING ADDICTION

If there is an "addictive personality," essentially it boils down to this: a belief that external substances, such as alcohol, to-bacco, cocaine, or heroin, are necessary to cope with, or get by in, life. Does either of the following sound familiar?

1. **Repeated attempts to prove that you are not addicted—that you can control, handle, or stop anytime at will.** If this were really the case, why would you need to prove it?
2. **A belief that you need the cigarette or the drink to function, or to handle stress, pressure, disappointments, or the variety of physical, emotional, or social discomforts that life, for better and worse, brings to us.** Everyone is stressed, but not everyone needs a substance like alcohol or cigarettes to get through the day. There is another way.

A key difference between alcoholism and smoking addiction is that although withdrawal from alcohol can be fatal, withdrawal from smoking is never fatal. If you are considering stopping drinking alcohol, work with a specialist or a hospital program to make sure you are safe through the period of withdrawal.

The National Council on Alcoholism and Drug Dependence also provides information about alcoholism and resources to help at: 244 East 58th Street, 4th Floor, New York, NY 10022. Phone: 212/269-7797. Fax: 212/269-7510. E-mail: national@ncadd.org. Web site: http://www.ncadd.org. Hope line: 800/NCA-CALL (24-hour affiliate referral).

The Situational Smoker

Like journalists on a deadline, these smokers turn to cigarettes when they feel intense pressure, or when they need to stay alert and finish a job. They then quit until the next high-pressure situation develops. Alternative patterns of nondaily situational smoking are associated with a variety of "off-duty" relaxing times and activities such as playing golf or meeting up with a friend. Research suggests that the following are typical triggers: relaxation, socializing, eating, drinking alcohol, and negative affect (Shiffman and Paty, *Journal of Abnormal Psychology*, August, 2006). These occasional bouts of smoking, however, sometimes become conditioned to a specific time or place where smokers appear to grant themselves "permission" to smoke. Situational smokers often behave like incomplete quitters who strain to stay smoke-free: unlike the recreational smoker, they are never completely at ease and free from the compulsion to smoke. These occasional bouts of smoking sometimes become conditioned to a specific time or place but can also become more generalized to other times and places. .

Patrick R. was a burly Irish-American with an outgoing personality, a demanding job in publishing, and a busy family life. He didn't smoke all weekend, but Monday morning in the office was his trigger and his green light to "smoke just one." He would take frequent smoking breaks throughout the day, huddling outside the building's entrance with his cigarette in hand. In the past, colleagues used to join him, but now there were few other smokers at the company, so his smoking had become a solitary, rather than a social, occurrence.

He never understood his office smoking. It was just an ingrained, automatic habit. Perhaps looking for reasons was part of his problem: he felt he could stop once he understood why he smoked, but since he couldn't figure it out, he never stopped smoking. However, he had some serious health worries, and a family history of heart disease, smoking, and early death. He was suspicious that even if he did quit, and overcame his "dark secret," he might die young anyway. Still, he was troubled by the hold smoking had on him.

Eventually, he admitted that he occasionally would have a cigarette or cigar on the weekend when he went to the store for the newspaper or at his golf club if he had a drink. So, in fact, "situational smokers" may not be so restricted to one place and one cigarette at a time after all.

"Situational smokers" believe they are in control of their smoking and are not really addicted. After all, they stop for long stretches of time on weekends or vacations when spending time with their family. They are sure no one in the family even knows they smoke. However, they still want to quit because they are ashamed and don't want their spouse or children to find out they smoke. They worry about their health as well.

Since it is normal for them to stop for periods of time, they are confident that even if they smoke, they can always stop whenever they want. This is the kind of faulty logic that perpetuates their periodic smoking. Called the "slot machine syndrome" because the payoff is irregular, this behavior is hard to extinguish. These are not recreational smokers, although they may appear to be. The difference is the regular, driven, involuntary, "out-of-control" nature of "situational smokers" ' behavior, even if it is tied to only certain places and situations.

What Kind of Smoker Are You?

It is possible, of course, that you fit into more than one category. If this is the case, you will have to make an extra effort compared with someone who fits into only one. Try not to focus on the injustice of having to do more than a hypothetical person you are imagining who has it so much easier. Comparing yourself with others will keep you stuck in resentment when what you need is to get moving and be productive. Facing hardships, like smoking addiction, can also bring unexpected lifelong benefits, such as emotional self-confidence and self-reliance, and a sense that you can handle life's problems when they come your way.

In this chapter, you have been introduced to different types of smokers. Which one or ones apply to you?

Recreational or Social Smoker
Scared-to-Quit Smoker
Emotion-Triggered Smoker
Worried-about-Weight Smoker
Alcoholic Smoker
Situational Smoker

Keeping a journal is a useful way to chart your progress in your efforts to quit. I explain in detail in "Your Smoke-Free 30-Day Calendar" (Part IV) how to do this. For now, use a notebook that will serve as your journal later to write up the story of your smoking, taking the stories of the types of smoker described in this chapter as a model. In the next section you'll find out which obstacles to quitting apply to the kind or kinds of smoker you are.

As you begin to decide how you want to quit, it is useful to consider some of the obstacles you will need to overcome, depending on the kind of smoker you are. If you've tried to quit before, these may be familiar to you, and may be where you got stuck in the past.

Obstacles to Quitting for Each Kind of Smoker

Obstacles to becoming smoke-free can vary for each type of smoker.

- If you are a **Recreational or Social Smoker,** you may feel that your limited smoking poses no serious medical harm to yourself or others. You may, however, ignore warning signs that your occasional smoking is progressing into addiction, especially during periods of stress or increased alcohol use. A periodic review of these warning signs (see pages 116, 118, and 129) may help motivate you to consider becoming smoke-free.

- The **Scared-to-Quit Smoker** has no end of reasons (excuses) to put off going smoke-free to some future date. Sometimes it helps to focus on just quitting for one day. If you can quit for a day, you can quit every day. This realization can be a great confidence builder, and helps to decrease your fears about not smoking "ever again." Forever is too big a word for many addicts; thus the old adage "Take it a day at a time." Just try to make each and every smoke-free day a good one!

- The **Emotion-Triggered Smoker** believes he or she needs the cigarette to handle life's big and small problems. Once the emotional trigger to smoke becomes more conscious, you can use this awareness as a tool. Remember: if every time you have gotten angry for 20 years, you have taken a cigarette, this impulse will

not vanish overnight. Wanting a cigarette will not hurt
you. Human beings have all kinds of thoughts and
feelings that in themselves are harmless if not put into
action. If you are an emotion-triggered smoker, you
need to keep your thoughts and feelings about smoking
in the realm of your mind and not act on them. There
is a saying: Don't just do something, sit there. Let the
feeling pass without smoking, and you'll find over time
that you can cope with it better than you ever imagined!

- The **Worried-about-Weight Smoker** may be trying
to live up to standards that breed dissatisfaction and
discontent. Start by trying to decrease worries about
weight rather than trying to lose it! The obstacle here
may be fear of making a "reasonable compromise." Yes,
you may gain a few pounds, but you'll do so much to
improve your health. In life we often have a choice
about how we wish to view a situation. Worrying about
weight may keep you from considering other elements
in your situation. Focus on other important realities,
such as preserving your family life or your physical
well-being or finding other (more creative and new)
ways to increase your metabolism—like interval walking
(alternating the speed of your pace). The confidence
gained from becoming smoke-free will help you find
new solutions to old problems, like weight, down the
road.

- The **Alcoholic Smoker** needs to distinguish between
good guilt and shame and bad guilt and shame. Bad
guilt and shame can paralyze you because of actions
(or inactions) you may have taken in the past which
hurt others or yourself. It is a counterproductive form
of self-punishment. Good guilt can lead you to examine
past actions, take stock of yourself, and learn to be

the person you wish you had been all along. With bad
guilt, you don't forgive yourself for your alcoholism; you
just feel bad about it. With good guilt, you can learn to
forgive yourself and to live with your imperfections even
as you dedicate yourself to trying to make changes in
your life.

- The **Situational Smoker** is different from the other
kinds of smokers described above. In each of the other
types (except the truly Recreational Smoker, who is not
addicted), the smoker comes to realize that he or she
has lost control over smoking (see below), and that
stopping completely is the only way to get back the lost
control. Because these situational smokers stop relatively
easily for periods of time, they never really believe they
have lost control and thereby lose a powerful motivation
for going smoke-free. They search for reasons why
they smoke, as if these will spontaneously cure them,
when mostly this fruitless search just perpetuates their
situation.

Focusing on this smoking pattern as a product of pure
behavioral conditioning may be more productive than
searching for reasons you smoke. Once you stop smoking
completely you'll discover your triggers and can eliminate
them from your life or learn to cope with them in new ways,
without smoking. In the meantime, while you are still trying
to quit, avoiding places associated with smoking conditioning can help enormously. Recent laws against smoking in
offices, restaurants, and bars in many parts of the country
make this easier.

REALIZING YOU'VE LOST CONTROL

With the exception of the Recreational Smoker, all the smokers described in this chapter share the experience of losing control over their smoking behavior. Realizing that you've lost control can become both the first step in, and an important motivator for, becoming smoke-free. What exactly does acknowledging "loss of control" do to help you prepare to quit? This step is like the first step for the alcoholic, who has to admit or accept he or she is an alcoholic before being able to get help. You need to take the idea of smoking addiction seriously enough to be willing to make a radical change in your smoking behavior: to throw away your cigarettes for good.

Although cigarettes are firmly in control of your behavior, you may be hung up on proving that you, not the cigarettes, are in charge. This is a fruitless battle, and step one is designed to help you face this reality.

Like an old boxer who is getting beaten to a pulp every time he enters the ring, addicted smokers succumb each time to the compulsion to smoke. The only power they have is to leave, to say good-bye, as in any abusive relationship.

Many smokers believe they have control over their smoking when they don't. This is one more of the false beliefs that keep them locked into their smoking addiction. There is great power in submitting to reality. Recognizing our limits is not a defeat but a starting point for cooperating successfully with the world, in this case giving up a losing battle to control smoking addiction, in the hope of becoming a recreational smoker!

Part II

PREPARING TO QUIT

CHAPTER 3

Deciding How You Want to Stop

You've learned by now that addiction has both behavioral and biological components. It's important to consider how you want to address both of these aspects. This chapter gives you the story of how one person decided. Through his example, you can see the range of choices you have available. It's up to you to decide if you want to use medication to help you stop smoking, but if you do use one of the medications discussed in this chapter and in Chapter 4, remember that it is only one part of a full plan that includes behavioral changes as well.

Dave G., a graphic designer, had tried to stop smoking several times before he came to see me, but was not very successful. He would cut down, making a note of each cigarette he smoked, but then he would return to smoking "three packs on a good day, four on a bad one." His wife was so concerned about his smoking that she contacted me about his serious addiction and asked me if I could help him.

On our first meeting, Dave told me that he enjoyed the first smoke of the day, but it was downhill from there. He told me, "I'm tired of not going places where I can't smoke; it limits my life." He had clearly lost the battle for control, and his world was closing in on him, leaving him feeling alone with his cigarettes.

Dave had a number of problems that made it especially hard for him to quit. He was a recovering alcoholic who had been sober for 11 years and had overcome a dependency on prescription medication. He also suffered from bipolar disorder and agoraphobia, a fear of being in public places. And he had occasional, painful bouts of depression and panic attacks. If NRT worked for him as a bridge out of smoking, imagine how it might work for you, especially if you don't have the many complications Dave had to face.

Since Dave used NRT to quit, this is a good point to introduce NRT—what it is, what it does, and what it doesn't do.

Concerns about Nicotine Replacement Therapy (NRT)

Many smokers are more afraid of the nicotine patch and other forms of NRT than they are of cigarettes. This makes no real sense, since cigarettes kill, and NRT has been proved safe over decades of use.

You might find it puzzling that you can take nicotine to get over nicotine addiction, and you may wonder if this is just replacing one addiction with another. At the end of this chapter I share with you a conversation I had with one of the world's foremost experts on nicotine, Jack Henningfield.

Dr. Henningfield has been a leader in helping us understand the difference between using pure nicotine as a medicine to stop smoking versus using it in the toxic cocktail known as the modern cigarette.

Because NRT is a powerful tool to help smokers quit, I want to urge you to read this chapter carefully. You'll see that there are no major or lasting risks associated with the proper use of NRT, and that this method can put you on the road to being smoke-free painlessly and without risks to your health.

NRT DOES NOT:
- Cause cancer!
- Go into your lungs!
- Prolong nicotine withdrawal!
- Make you more likely to return to smoking!

NRT DOES:
- Make it easier to stop smoking!

The Key to Finding the Right Dose

The biggest problem with NRT is that people just don't use it correctly. There are some key points about how best to use each kind of NRT to get the most out of it. Dave's experience offers some pitfalls to beware of.

When he came to see me, Dave had previously tried NRT, but it had not worked, in large part because the dose he used was too low. We discussed an aggressive NRT strategy. Remember, it is called "nicotine replacement" for a reason, and he was a big smoker, so he needed a larger-than-usual dose.

Another problem with his previous attempts to quit was his use of NRT to cut down. Some people can back out of smoking this way, but in Dave's case, he began using NRT to try to control, not stop, smoking. We needed to address these two problems in his new quit plan—focusing on accepting not smoking at all, and increasing the amount of NRT he would use.

The goal of NRT is to replace your daily nicotine intake in a safe form. The best way to accomplish this is to remember that approximately 1 mg of nicotine is absorbed for each cigarette smoked. If you smoke a pack a day, you have to replace those 20 cigarettes with approximately 20 mg of nicotine. Dave was smoking 60 to 80 cigarettes a day, so he needed 60 to 80 mg of nicotine per day. I therefore recommended that he start with two 21-mg nicotine patches (see page 51) and use a nicotine oral inhaler as needed (see page 55).

This might seem like a lot of nicotine, but it was still less than the total amount of nicotine he had been getting from smoking. Plus, it would be pure nicotine, without all the poisons and chemicals found in tobacco smoke. Medically, he would be 1 million times safer just switching from smoking to NRT, and it would provide him with hope and a bridge out of smoking. I explained that *NRT works to heal the addiction only when you quit smoking completely*. It may help short-term to control the addiction, or to prepare for a quit day while you are still smoking (see page 82), but the key to successfully quitting with NRT is to use it as a substitute for, not a complement to, smoking. I explained that if you smoke even just a little after your quit day, it is like feeding a beast that will only want more. On the other hand, if you go completely smoke-free, you will be starving the beast, and healing physically and mentally from the addiction. Even if you have discomfort (either from things going on in your life, or from cigarette withdrawal), it is discomfort for a good cause. Living through this discomfort can help you to heal from the addiction to cigarettes and find new ways to handle your life without smoking.

How to Use the Various Forms of NRT

The following descriptions of medications to help stop smoking are brief and general in nature. If you are pregnant, breastfeeding, or have a serious medical illness, it is always a good idea to discuss your plans to take a smoking cessation medication with your doctor. For more information you can also check the medication guide created by the Tobacco Control Research Branch of the National Cancer Institute: http://www.smokefree.gov/quit-smoking/medicationguide/ or http://www.smokefree.gov/.

NICOTINE PATCH

This popular NRT delivery system comes in a few standard doses.

- 21 mg delivered and absorbed (approximately equivalent of 21 cigarettes a day)
- 14 mg delivered and absorbed (approximately equivalent of 14 cigarettes a day)
- 7 mg delivered and absorbed (approximately equivalent of 7 cigarettes a day)

Instructions for Use: The 21-mg patch replaces approximately a pack per day. Use the 14-mg or 7-mg patch for tapering off, or 10 or fewer cigarettes a day. Apply a new patch daily on a clean, dry, non-hairy upper body site. Use only after smoking cessation. Taper off over 8 weeks, and you feel confident in your smoke-free lifestyle.

Advantages: Easy to use.

Side Effects: A rash is common, so be sure to rotate the patch site daily. Remove the patch before bed if you experience disturbed sleep. Side effects may include: Headaches, dizziness/lightheadedness, drowsiness and stomach-upset/nausea. **Always follow package directions. For detailed product information go to:** http://habitrol.com/product.html or http://www.nicodermcq.com/.

NICOTINE GUM

This is another popular NRT delivery system that comes in smaller standard doses.

- 2 mg: 2 mg delivered; approximately 1 mg absorbed, the equivalent of 1 cigarette
- 4 mg: 4 mg delivered; approximately 2 mg absorbed, the equivalent of 2 cigarettes

Instructions for Use: Do not chew like ordinary gum! Nicotine is absorbed through the inside of your mouth (buccal mucosa). Alternate chewing (until tingling feeling or peppery taste in mouth) and "parking" between cheek and gums. The 4-mg gum is most effective if you smoke 24 or more cigarettes. Ten pieces of nicotine gum replace a pack a day (approximately 20 mg absorbed). One important note about nicotine gum: regular preventive use (for example, a piece or two every hour) is more effective than simply taking it "as needed" when the urge arises. By that point, it may be too late, since a little time is required for the nicotine to enter your system. Tapering schedule is usually over 3 months. Acidic beverages (coffee, tea, citrus juices, sodas) inactivate nicotine; do not consume them during or for 15 minutes before active gum use.

Side effects: May include a bad taste from the gum; tingling feeling on tongue when chewing gum; hiccups; upset stomach; nausea, heartburn; jaw pain caused by chewing. Side effects are often associated with excess nicotine in the mouth from chewing like regular gum (not "parking" or waiting after a few chews for inside the mouth absorption to occur). Chewing too fast can cause: lightheadedness, dizziness, hiccups, nausea, vomiting, and insomnia. **Always follow package directions. For detailed product information go to:** http://www.gsk-scrc.com/products/default.aspx.

NICOTINE LOZENGE

Similar to nicotine gum, the lozenge offers smaller doses of nicotine throughout the day.

- 2 mg: 2 mg delivered; approximately 1 mg absorbed (equivalent of 1 cigarette)
- 4 mg; 4 mg delivered; approximately 2 mg absorbed (equivalent of 2 cigarettes)

Instructions for Use: Allow the lozenge to dissolve slowly in your mouth over 20 to 30 minutes in order to deliver the labeled amount of nicotine, half of which is absorbed by your body. Dosing and the way the body absorbs the nicotine in the lozenge are exactly the same as for gum. Chewing, biting, or swallowing renders the nicotine in the lozenge less effective, as it is inactivated by stomach acid. Likewise, acidic beverages inactivate the nicotine in the lozenge and should be avoided for 15 minutes before and while the lozenge is in your mouth.

Advantages: The lozenge is helpful for those who want an oral medication but do not like to chew gum. Decreased weight gain is also reported for the duration of use.

Side Effects: May include soreness of teeth and gums, indigestion, irritated throat. **Always follow package directions. For detailed product information go to:** http://www.commitlozenge.com/.

NICOTINE NASAL SPRAY

By prescription only:

- 1 spray in each nostril results in 1 mg delivered (and approximately 0.5 mg absorbed by the body), the equivalent of a half a cigarette. Forty doses replace approximately a pack a day.

Instructions for Use: The nicotine spray is absorbed faster than other forms of NRT. You can taper off the nasal spray over 4 to 6 weeks by skipping doses. Recommended use is 3 to 6 months.

Advantages: The spray is absorbed faster than other forms of nicotine replacement, and so is most useful to people with strong and sudden cravings that may portend a relapse into smoking.

Side Effects: May include sneezing, coughing, and watering eyes. Tolerance to these effects can occur in the first week. **Always follow package directions. For detailed product**

information go to: http://www.pfizer.com/products/rx/rx
_product_nicotrol.jsp.

NICOTINE ORAL INHALER

By prescription only:

- 10-mg cartridge: 4 mg delivered; approximately 2 mg
  absorbed by your body, the approximate equivalent of
  2 cigarettes

Instructions for Use: You can take 80 puffs over 20 to 30 minutes. This delivers 4 mg of nicotine (approximately 2 mg absorbed) to the mouth and throat (none of the nicotine goes
to the lungs). Ten cartridges replace approximately 1 pack
a day (approximately 20 mg absorbed). The best results are
achieved with frequent puffing. For maximum effectiveness,
as with nicotine gum and the lozenge, do not consume
acidic beverages (coffee, tea, citrus juices, sodas) for 15
minutes before or while puffing on the inhaler. Cold winter
air can interfere with nicotine delivery, so consider more frequent puffing in colder weather. You can taper off the oral
inhaler over 4 to 6 weeks by skipping doses. Recommended
use up to 6 months. The manufacturer suggests an upper
limit of 16 cartridges of nicotine oral inhaler per day.
Advantages: The inhaler has the hand-to-mouth feel of cigarettes, and like the gum, it can serve as a substitute ritual for
smoking.
Side effects: May include mouth and throat irritation and
coughing. Smokers with respiratory problems should use
with caution. **Always follow package directions. For detailed product information go to:** http://www.pfizer.com/
products/rx/rx_product_nicotrol.jsp.

GETTING THE FULL BENEFITS OF NRT

Although NRT is a major advance in helping smokers quit, it can be used even more effectively if the following are kept in mind:

- Make sure the dose is not too low.
- Make sure of your motivation in using NRT: is it to control your addiction to smoking (for a plane ride or a meeting for example) or to quit completely?
- Be careful not to stop or cut down on NRT too soon. It is meant to be used for 8 to 12 weeks, or longer as needed, under the care of a doctor.
- Don't rely on NRT to do the whole job. It's important not to place all the burden on NRT. You must also be aware of other aspects of your addiction, besides the physical, which can affect your success. For example, if getting upset triggers a wish to smoke based on years of automated behavior, you will have to use your newfound understanding of your smoking addiction to interrupt these old, repetitive patterns. Although NRT makes it easier, you have to take advantage of this by addressing your personal behavioral and emotional triggers as well.

Maximizing the Effectiveness of NRT

Remember Dave, our recovering alcoholic smoker at the beginning of this chapter? In addition to NRT, he implemented a number of lifestyle changes that were equally important to his overall quit plan. I discussed with Dave the need to use deep, slow breathing to calm and distract himself if, and when, he had urges and cravings to smoke. I recommended he drink water, and carry a water bottle, as a new ritual to help distract him from the empty hunger-like pangs of withdrawal. We also discussed the importance of avoiding other smokers. Dave said this would be easy for him, since he was pretty much the last smoker in his social circle.

We set a specific quit date to make the quit plan "real" and take the addiction out of the shadows where it likes to live. I emphasized the difference between quitting completely and for good versus trying to bargain with the addiction by controlling when and where you smoke. When you try to control the addiction, it keeps the upper hand; when you stop smoking completely, you can get on with your life without smoking.

The Quit Day and Beyond

Dave did not smoke at all on his quit day, and he reported that it was "easier than I thought it would be." He said, however, that at one point on the day after his quit day he felt like smoking when he got upset, but didn't. Day two was more difficult than day one, yet he was still not smoking. He was using two patches plus a nicotine oral inhaler; he was also drinking water and breathing deeply and slowly to cope with cravings. He was changing the focus of his attention when craving, and this also helped him. He said he felt threatened by smokers in the street and was avoiding them. He was thinking of smoke-free environments to spend time in over the weekend.

The week following his quit date, Dave reported no smoking for 8 days! On day nine it was tougher; he was more anxious, especially when he traveled farther from his home. A voice in his head kept telling him he was "too weak to succeed" at not smoking. He began to see how getting upset triggered the wish to smoke. On the positive side, though, he was thinking about large and small things to look forward to as a nonsmoker.

When he told me he had cut down on using the nicotine oral inhaler, because he was feeling successful, I suggested that he use the nicotine oral inhaler more, and that he should view success as coming from his efforts—not as a matter of luck or of being weak or strong. We discussed the need to disconnect the automatic response between getting upset and smoking.

The Role of NRT Later
in the Quitting Process

At 3 weeks, Dave reported no smoking for 21 days! He was finding this "easier than feared." He was using the patches and inhaler as directed. He was more aware now of his nerves and anxiety, as well as his sadness and anger. He was concerned with the need for something to do with his hands, and we discussed puzzles and knitting (yes, a lot of men like to knit), two things he enjoyed. His skin looked markedly better, and he reported fewer thoughts about smoking.

At 4 weeks, he again reported no smoking. He said it was getting better and easier. Because he still felt out of shape and out of breath, he decided to start walking and stretching. He was less anxious and withdrawn and his agoraphobia was better. At the same time he was aware of feeling more depressed and felt he was having a "midlife crisis" about what to do with his life. Overall, he was getting more comfortable in his reality as a nonsmoker. He would stick with his NRT regimen for another week, and then we would discuss whether it was time to taper off.

By week 5, he still reported no smoking. In general he said he was having no cravings, but his thoughts about smoking went up and down and he didn't feel ready to taper off NRT yet. He was looking into a trainer and a gym. He said he was enjoying going out more and spending some time in the country.

At 6 weeks and beyond, Dave continued to build on his new nonsmoking life. He was beginning an exercise program, and had a personal trainer. He wanted to lose 7 pounds and was trying a new diet. He reported an increase in feelings of mourning for his father, who had died of lung cancer, and he had put up his father's picture at home. He said he was much less withdrawn, and felt more alert. He was pursuing some creative work that interested him.

Dave still reported cravings when he saw people smoking, and also when he experienced strong anxious emotions. But he was learning to cope and adjust without tobacco. He wanted to reinforce the feeling that he could have a good and creative life and cope well without smoking. He was isolating himself less, connecting more with friends, getting exercise, and looking forward to new projects.

Dave didn't feel comfortable tapering off his NRT until he had not smoked for 84 days! The plan was now to taper off over the next 2 weeks to 14-mg patches, and to monitor how he was doing. He felt he no longer needed so much nicotine by this point. Most of his triggers to smoke had faded. He was not thinking about smoking. He could still get moody, but felt more emotionally stable. He was also no longer agoraphobic, was more social, and in general felt he was headed down a "good track."

KEY POINT

Don't rush tapering off NRT. Some people take forever to stop smoking and then want to stop the NRT as soon as possible. Dave knew when he felt confident and on a good track, and that's when he began to slowly taper off the NRT.

FOLLOW-UP 5 YEARS LATER

Dave reported he was not smoking after 5 years! He felt the "NRT was 50 percent of what helped me, along with the behavioral things." He said he was working, less isolated, and more engaged with life.

Although NRT is designed to be used as a helpful tool, it can't carry the whole burden of treating smoking addiction. Changing your mental attitude and using your heightened self-awareness of smoking triggers (see pages 115 and 137–38) will help you get the most out of therapies like the gum, patch, and oral inhaler.

A LEADING EXPERT ANSWERS QUESTIONS ABOUT NRT

Dr. Jack Henningfield has been a pioneer in helping us understand addictive drugs and in developing medications for the treatment of addictions. He has taken a special interest in nicotine and tobacco research. Following are Dr. Henningfield's answers to the questions I know are most often on the minds of smokers considering NRT.

DOES THE NICOTINE IN NRT CAUSE CANCER OR HEART ATTACKS?

Nicotine has been thoroughly evaluated for its potential role in cancer and heart disease. In the form of nicotine replacement therapy (NRT), the nicotine is in a relatively low dose and pure form as compared with cigarettes and other tobacco products.

There is no evidence that nicotine medications cause heart attacks or cancer, or contribute to other forms of heart disease. In fact, the most recent report of the International Agency for Research on Cancer (2004) did not list nicotine among the carcinogens in tobacco. In the form of tobacco products, however, nicotine is typically delivered much more rapidly and at much higher dosages than nicotine from NRT products. And in tobacco products, the nicotine is delivered in the form of deadly chemical cocktails. For example, one of the components of cigarette smoke is carbon monoxide, which has well-established toxic effects on the heart; carbon monoxide exposure can contribute to a heart attack. It is possible that the effects of the explosively high doses of nicotine delivered by inhaling tobacco smoke would add to the effects of carbon monoxide and other substances.

HOW CAN YOU TAKE NICOTINE TO GET OVER NICOTINE ADDICTION?

The high addiction risk of cigarettes is due to their high-speed delivery of large doses of nicotine and their engineering to increase the risk of addiction. For example, a high-dose nicotine patch delivers about 1 mg of nicotine to the body per hour, and the use of nicotine gum typically results in absorption of about 1 to 2 mg over 20 to 30 minutes for each dose that is used. A cigarette can easily deliver 1 to 3 mg of nicotine within a few minutes of smoking, with high spiking blood levels occurring within the first few puffs. Furthermore, cigarette smoke is a complex chemical cocktail with many substances and design features to increase its addictiveness. Thus, substituting an NRT product for cigarettes immediately replaces the high-dose chemical cocktail with lower and controlled dosages of pure nicotine. In addition, the instructions for use ("labeling") for the NRT products have been designed to minimize the risk of addiction and provide guidance for termination of drug use when it is no longer needed. The NRT product does partially substitute for the addictive actions of nicotine and does provide some of the effects that can contribute to addiction, such as helping to control mood, maintain concentration, and minimize stress. This provides the equivalent of a gentle cushion, relative to cigarettes, so that the person attempting to achieve and maintain freedom from tobacco can accomplish the goal.

CAN I GET NICOTINE POISONING FROM NRT— FOR EXAMPLE, FROM THE PATCH?

Nicotine is a potent drug and that is why the Food and Drug Administration carefully restricts the amount of nicotine that is contained in the products and sets limits on the allowable amounts that can be taken per day. Follow the package directions and make sure that the dose you select is right for you (e.g., high doses of nicotine patches should be used only by people who smoke more than 10 cigarettes per day, and the high-dose nicotine lozenge should be used only by people who smoke their first cigarette within 30 minutes upon waking each day). Exceeding the labeled instructions can result in effects such as dizziness, nausea, and even intoxication. There have been no known cases of overdose deaths resulting from the use of NRT products.

I HEARD THAT NICOTINE IS OUT OF YOUR SYSTEM IN 2 TO 3 DAYS. HOW LONG IS NICOTINE WITHDRAWAL? IS IT THE SAME FOR EVERYONE?

Nicotine delivery to the body causes the physically addicting changes in the brain that drive compulsive tobacco use. These changes include adaptive changes (such as increased brain nicotine receptors) that help the body tolerate this high-dose invasion of nicotine. Then, when nicotine administration stops, the body rebounds in many ways: heart rate slows, brain waves that were suppressed become more active, calm is replaced by nervousness, and so on. For most people these and other withdrawal symptoms are worst for the first few days and taper off over about a month or so.

In part, NRT works by preventing the body from abruptly going from very high daily nicotine to zero. This provides the equivalent of a controlled cushion for the body and allows the person to learn to live without cigarettes as the nicotine levels are gradually reduced, generally over a few months. The strength, nature, and duration of the withdrawal vary widely across people, however. For example, severe depression and strong feelings of anger occur in some people, whereas for others an inability to concentrate is the main problem. For some people, a powerful craving for a cigarette can be triggered by the smell of smoke or sight of cigarettes for many months after the physical withdrawal seems to have pretty much run its course. For these reasons, smoking cessation is viewed as a long-term process for most people; and because the individual may not know how long the withdrawal will last, everyone should quit smoking with a plan and support as needed.

CHAPTER 4

Do You Need a Doctor to Quit?

As we discussed in Chapter 3, there are two kinds of NRT: one available without a prescription, and the other (which includes the inhaler and spray) that requires a prescription. If you decide that you are interested in the inhaler or nasal spray, you need to talk with your doctor, dentist, or nurse practitioner.

But even if you don't need a prescription from your doctor, it's still worth discussing NRT with him or her. Your doctor can be an ally, and a person to report to about how it's going for you. The doctor may also have his or her own way of motivating you, based on your particular medical situation and on the doctor's knowledge of you as a person.

If you decide to use NRT, you and your doctor can decide if prescription forms will be helpful to you. Some insurance plans (including Medicaid) will cover NRT like the patch and the gum, so check with your plan to see if a prescription can lower your costs. (A review of all the forms of NRT can be found in "Day Two" of the "Your Smoke-Free 30-Day Calendar." And your doctor can also help you figure out if the two medications discussed in this chapter—Zyban and Chantix—might be right for you.

Some doctors give out prescriptions for NRT to help stop smoking without any initial counseling or supportive follow-up. However, just relying on a prescription often doesn't address the fear-based avoidance behavior so common among smokers. Many doctors also needlessly exaggerate the difficulty of nicotine withdrawal, which for many smokers is, fortunately, not as bad as the way it is often presented. A story in the *Wall Street Journal* emphasized the horror of withdrawal depression using the phrase "nicotine's dark and powerful grip on the brain." This story line also plays into the smoker's rationale for continued smoking: "You see, even doctors say physical withdrawal has a powerful grip."

Just giving a prescription to a frightened smoker can be like asking people who don't know how to swim, and are afraid to try, to jump off the high diving board. They just won't do it! Smokers need the confidence to try, and they need to believe they can be successful. They need to believe that their life can and will be better, not worse, without smoking. Thankfully, this is almost always the case when smokers follow through with the *Smoke-Free in 30 Days* program.

Common Medication Strategies

Below is information for you to review with your prescriber on common medication strategies. In brief, they are bupropion (Zyban, Wellbutrin) alone; bupropion plus NRT (patch, gum, or inhaler); and varenicline (Chantix). The following descriptions of medications to help stop smoking are brief and general in nature. If you are pregnant, breastfeeding, or have a serious medical illness, it is always a good idea to discuss your plans to take a smoking cessation medication with your doctor. For more information you can also check the medication guide created by the Tobacco Control Research Branch of the National Cancer Institute: http://www.smokefree.gov/quit smoking/medicationguide/ or http://www.smokefree.gov/.

BUPROPION

Bupropion (Zyban, Wellbutrin) is available by prescription only. For bupropion, the best dose for smoking cessation is 300 mg/day.

Instructions for Use: Plan to start taking bupropion 7 to 10 days before you intend to stop smoking. It can be good to start with 100-mg or 150-mg tablets and then increase to 300-mg tablets. If you use 150-mg tablets, these must be taken 8 hours apart (often, 10 AM and 6 PM are good).

Never double up if a dose is missed. Use for 7 to 12 weeks or longer as your doctor advises until cessation is successful and you have confidence in a smoke-free lifestyle. Tapering off is not required. Bupropion works for both depressed and nondepressed individuals.

Advantages: Helpful for smokers who experience difficult moods after cessation or who have co-occurring elements of minor depression. Weight gain can be minimized during active use. It can be used alone or in combination with NRT.

Side Effects: Higher doses (above 300 mg/day) may be associated with seizures in some individuals, so Zyban is not recommended for smokers with a history of seizures, anorexia, alcohol dependence, or head trauma. Side effects may include: dry mouth, difficulty sleeping, headaches, dizziness, and skin rashes.

ZYBAN PLUS NRT

Zyban can be combined with nicotine replacement therapy to good effect.

Instructions for Use: 21-mg patches replace approximately a pack a day; 14-mg or 7-mg patches replace approximately about 10 or fewer cigarettes a day. See also the other NRT options, such as the gum and inhaler in Chapter 3. Take as directed by your doctor.

Side Effects: The American Cancer Society states: "This drug should not be taken if you have ever had seizures, heavy alcohol use, serious head injury, bipolar (manic-depressive) illness, anorexia or bulimia (eating disorders)." **Always follow package directions. For detailed product information go to:** www.glaxoSmithKline.com or http://us.gsk.com/products/assets/us_zyban.pdf.

CHANTIX

Chantix (varenicline) is available by prescription only.

Instructions for Use: It should be taken with food and started 1 week prior to the target quit date. Take 0.5 mg once daily for 3 days, then 0.5 mg twice daily for 4 days. Starting on the target quit date, take 1 mg twice daily for 11 weeks. If you're not smoking at the end of 12 weeks, you may continue on the advice of your doctor at 1 mg twice daily for an additional 12 weeks. You may stop Chantix abruptly; there is no need to taper off. Discuss potential side effects with your doctor.

Advantages: Easy to use, in pill form.

CHANTIX: SAFETY WARNINGS

Although there are advantages to the drug Chantix, there are some warnings that have been issued by the FDA and the Institute for Safe Medication Practices. According to the FDA, some serious neuropsychiatric symptoms have occurred in patients taking Chantix, including changes in behavior, agitation, depressed mood, suicidal ideation, and attempted and completed suicide. Please be sure to discuss possible side effects with your doctor. For more information, please see the FDA alert dated February 1, 2008, and the Institute for Safe Medication Practices report dated October 23, 2008. Visit www.fda .gov for the most up-to-date information about this and other drugs.

Side Effects: may include nausea, change in dreaming, constipation, gas and vomiting. Drowsiness can impair ability to drive or use machinery. Not known if it can be safely used in combination with bupropion or NRT. Smokers should not use varenicline if they have kidney problems. **Always follow package directions. For detailed product information go to:** http://www.chantix.com/.

Health Assessments to Take to Your Doctor

Some of us have more trouble quitting than others, and certain types of smokers may particularly benefit from NRT and close medical supervision while they are going smoke-free. If you have identified yourself in Chapter 2 as an Alcoholic Smoker or an Emotion-Triggered Smoker, please copy and fill out the assessments that follow, and make an appointment with your doctor to discuss medications *before* you begin the quitting process. These assessments can be a useful tool for your health care provider as well as for your own insight into your state of mind and level of addiction.

Your Depression Health Checkup

Do a self-assessment for depression. If it raises concerns, please show and discuss this self-assessment with your physician or a licensed mental health practitioner.

Thanks to Drs. Robert L. Spitzer, Kurt Kroenke, and Janet Williams for their permission to use the PHQ in our book.

PATIENT HEALTH QUESTIONNAIRE

This questionnaire is an important part of providing you with the best health care possible. Your answers will help in understanding problems that you may have. Please answer every question to the best of your ability unless you are requested to skip over a question.

Name _____ Age _____ Sex: ❏ Female ❏ Male
Today's Date _____

PHQ-9

Over the *last 2 weeks*, how often have you been bothered by any of the following problems?

(Use "✓" to indicate your answer)

	Not at all	Several days	More than half the days	Nearly every day
1. Little interest or pleasure in doing things	0	1	2	3
2. Feeling down, depressed, or hopeless	0	1	2	3
3. Trouble falling or staying asleep, or sleeping too much	0	1	2	3
4. Feeling tired or having little energy	0	1	2	3
5. Poor appetite or overeating	0	1	2	3
6. Feeling bad about yourself—or that you are a failure or have let yourself or your family down	0	1	2	3
7. Trouble concentrating on things, such as reading the newspaper or watching television	0	1	2	3

(*continued on next page*)

8. Moving or speaking so slowly that   0   1   2   3
    other people could have noticed. Or
    the opposite—being so fidgety or
    restless that you have been moving
    around a lot more than usual
9. Thoughts that you would be better   0   1   2   3
    off dead or of hurting yourself in
    some way

(For office coding: Total Score   _____ = _____ + _____ + _____)

If you checked off *any* problems, how *difficult* have these problems made it for you
to do your work, take care of things at home, or get along with other people?

Not difficult at all	Somewhat difficult	Very difficult	Extremely difficult
❏	❏	❏	❏

From the Primary Care Evaluation of Mental Disorders Patient Health Questionnaire (PRIME-MD PHQ). The PHQ was developed by Drs. Robert L. Spitzer, Janet B. W. Williams, Kurt Kroenke, and colleagues. For research information, contact Dr. Spitzer at ris8@columbia.edu.

ASSESSING YOUR DEPRESSION SCORE:

PHQ-9 Depression Severity. This is calculated by assigning scores of 0, 1, 2, and 3 to the response categories of "not at all," "several days," "more than half the days," and "nearly every day," respectively. PHQ-9 total score for the nine items ranges from 0 to 27. Scores of 5, 10, 15, and 20 represent cutpoints for mild, moderate, moderately severe, and severe depression, respectively. Sensitivity to change has also been confirmed.

PHQ-9 SCORES AND PROPOSED TREATMENT ACTIONS*

PHQ-9 Score	Depression Severity	Proposed Treatment Actions
0–4	None	None
5–9	Mild	Watchful waiting; repeat PHQ-9 at follow-up
10–14	Moderate	Treatment plan, considering counseling, follow-up and/or pharmacotherapy
15–19	Moderately Severe	Immediate initiation of pharmacotherapy and/or psychotherapy
20–27	Severe	Immediate initiation of pharmacotherapy and, if severe impairment or poor response to therapy, expedited referral to a mental health specialist for psychotherapy and/or collaborative management

* From K. Kroenke, R. L. Spitzer, *Psychiatric Annals,* 32 (2002): 509–521.

Your Anxiety Health Checkup

Do a self-assessment for anxiety. If it raises concerns, please show and discuss this self-assessment with your physician or a licensed mental health practitioner.

Thanks to Drs. Robert L. Spitzer, Kurt Kroenke, and Janet Williams for their permission to use the PHQ in our book.

PATIENT HEALTH QUESTIONNAIRE

This questionnaire is an important part of providing you with the best health care possible. Your answers will help in understanding problems that you may have. Please answer every question to the best of your ability unless you are requested to skip over a question.

Name _____ Age _____ Sex: ❏ Female ❏ Male
Today's Date _____

GAD-7

Over the *last 2 weeks*, how often have you been bothered by the following problems?

(Use "✓" to indicate your answer)

	Not at all	Several days	More than half the days	Nearly every day
1. Feeling nervous, anxious, or on edge	0	1	2	3
2. Not being able to stop or control worrying	0	1	2	3
3. Worrying too much about different things	0	1	2	3
4. Trouble relaxing	0	1	2	3
5. Being so restless that it is hard to sit still	0	1	2	3
6. Becoming easily annoyed or irritable	0	1	2	3
7. Feeling afraid as if something awful might happen	0	1	2	3

(*continued on next page*)

ASSESSING YOUR ANXIETY SCORE:

GAD-7 Anxiety Severity. This is calculated by assigning scores of 0, 1, 2, and 3 to the response categories of "not at all," "several days," "more than half the days," and "nearly every day," respectively. GAD-7 total score for the seven items ranges from 0 to 21. Scores of 5, 10, and 15 represent cutpoints for mild, moderate, and severe anxiety, respectively. Though designed primarily as a screening and severity measure for generalized anxiety disorder, the GAD-7 also has moderately good operating characteristics for three other common anxiety disorders—panic disorder, social anxiety disorder, and post-traumatic stress disorder. When screening for anxiety disorders, a recommended cutpoint for further evaluation is a score of 10 or greater.

Your Alcohol Health Checkup

Do a self-assessment for alcohol. If it raises concerns, please show and discuss this self-assessment with your physician or a licensed mental health practitioner.

Thanks to Drs. Robert L. Spitzer, Kurt Kroenke, and Janet Williams for their permission to use the PHQ in our book.

PATIENT HEALTH QUESTIONNAIRE

This questionnaire is an important part of providing you with the best health care possible. Your answers will help in understanding problems that you may have. Please answer every question to the best of your ability unless you are requested to skip over a question.

Name _____ Age _____ Sex: ❑ Female ❑ Male
Today's Date _____

		NO	YES
9.	Do you ever drink alcohol (including beer or wine)?	❑	❑

If you checked "NO" go to question #11.

10. Have any of the following happened to you *more than once in the last 6 months?*

	NO	YES
a. You drank alcohol even though a doctor suggested that you stop drinking because of a problem with your health	❑	❑
b. You drank alcohol, were high from alcohol, or hungover while you were working, going to school, or taking care of children or other responsibilities	❑	❑
c. You missed or were late for work, school, or other activities because you were drinking or hungover	❑	❑
d. You had a problem getting along with other people while you were drinking	❑	❑
e. You drove a car after having several drinks or after drinking too much	❑	❑

(*continued on next page*)

11. If you checked off *any* problems on this questionnaire, how *difficult* have these problems made it for you to do your work, take care of things at home, or get along with other people?

Not difficult at all	Somewhat difficult	Very difficult	Extremely difficult
❑	❑	❑	❑

Developed by Drs. Robert L. Spitzer, Janet B. W. Williams, Kurt Kroenke, and colleagues, with an educational grant from Pfizer Inc.

For research information, contact Dr. Spitzer at rls8@columbia.edu.

USING NRT *BEFORE* YOU QUIT? A NEW APPROACH TO DISCUSS WITH YOUR DOCTOR

The Australian government has recently approved a 21-mg patch for 2-week use before cessation—in other words, you use the patch to prepare for your quit day, rather than starting your NRT on the day you stop smoking. And other countries are following suit: in the United Kingdom, after an extensive review of the safety data,* there is no longer a warning against smoking while using 2-mg nicotine gum, 4-mg nicotine gum, and the nicotine oral inhaler. Instead, in the United Kingdom, some NRT products are licensed to cut down smoking as a stepping-stone to stopping completely, for smokers who are currently unable to stop abruptly.

Despite the widespread belief among smokers and doctors that smoking while using the patch and other forms of NRT can cause nicotine overdose and heart attacks, there is a growing body of credible research that contradicts this belief. New studies also suggest that smoking while on the patch, for a maximum period of 2 weeks, with a clear goal of ending smoking completely on a specific date, can enhance the ability of smokers to have a successful quit day.

This approach has now been recognized with a name: "pre-quit treatment with nicotine patch." A general overview of this approach[†] found it to "double the odds of quitting" and has the potential to be an innovative way to use NRT to help smokers quit. This overview also states that all the studies done so far reported no safety issues in using the pre-quit treatment with nicotine patch (PQNP).

However, because this research is relatively new and limited in scope, using NRT before you quit was not endorsed by the most recent (2008) U.S. government guidelines on "Treating Tobacco Use and Dependence." These guidelines do, however, provide advice to smokers who may choose to try NRT before they quit. They state: "If this strategy is used clinically, patients should be advised to cease NRT use if they develop symptoms of nicotine toxicity (e.g., nausea, vomiting, dizziness)."

Even though you can purchase the nicotine patch at a pharmacy without a prescription, be sure to carefully review your PQNP plan with a physician, dentist, nurse practitioner, or knowledgeable tobacco cessation specialist. Keep in mind that smoking while on the patch is not an FDA-approved treatment in the United States.

Note of caution: While this approach may give you a running start on your quit day, don't expect the patch to do all the work necessary for your long-term success. As I stress repeatedly, while NRT is a helpful tool, it is not meant to carry the whole burden of making this important change in your life.

* Committee on Safety of Medicines and Healthcare Products Regulatory Agency (CSMHPRA). *Report on the Committee on Safety of Medicines Working Group on Nicotine Replacement Therapy* (London: CSM and MHRSA, 2006). Available at http://www.mhra.gov.uk.

† See Saul Shiffman and Stuart G. Ferguson, "Nicotine Patch Therapy Prior to Quitting Smoking: A Meta-Analysis," *Addiction*, 103, 4 (March 13, 2008): 557–563. Published online.

CHAPTER 5

What Will Your Last Week as a Smoker Be Like?

Many smokers mistakenly believe that smoking is a uniquely wonderful experience (or at least they believed this when they started). But in fact, once they honestly examine the day-to-day truth about their smoking, most smokers acknowledge that it isn't wonderful at all anymore, even though it is (or once was) associated with such enjoyable experiences as drinking alcohol and coffee, going to parties or bars, and sex. In order to quit, it is necessary to change your behavior and separate smoking from these other activities. As we've seen, smoking can also be linked to negative emotional states, such as anger and depression, and it is necessary to break that link as well. Both positive and negative triggers have to be decoupled from smoking in order for you to succeed in going smoke-free.

The goal is to stop the internal war between the part of you that wants to smoke and the part of you that wants to quit, and learn to make a lasting peace. This happens as you build your commitment to change, and work your way through the series of confidence-building exercises.

Smoking by the Clock

One of the most effective pre-quit techniques I suggest to my patients is called "smoking by the clock." Approximately 1 week before our target quit date, I put my patients on a strict smoking schedule. Spending a week smoking on schedule is a short-term way to help you prepare for the day you will go tobacco-free altogether. The object is to "smoke by the clock," in other words, by adhering to a carefully constructed smoking schedule. This means you smoke your cigarettes on schedule—whether you want to or not. If you smoke only when you want to smoke, you will merely reinforce old patterns and habits. By literally scheduling your smoking, you are interrupting these automatic behaviors. This prepares the ground for change.

Start by counting the number of cigarettes you smoke each day. Then count the numbers of hours you are awake each day. For example, if you are awake 18 hours a day (starting at 8 AM) and you smoke 18 cigarettes a day, you would smoke your first cigarette at 8 AM. If you miss an hour, do not double up later. Remember: once you make the schedule, stick with it! The purpose of this exercise is to begin to wean yourself, not from actual cigarettes just yet, but from your usual *triggers* (situations, thoughts, or feelings) connected with smoking. We want to help take you off automatic pilot and begin to interrupt these patterns so you can shed them on the day you choose to become completely tobacco-free.

One more key to success with this exercise: don't try to cut down on the number of cigarettes you smoke each day at this point; just stick to your schedule so that you can't smoke anytime you want to—you can smoke only when the clock tells you it's time. For now, surrender to the clock! If you are a situational smoker, smoke by the clock only during your usual smoking times and in your usual places.

Other Ways to Change Your Behavior before Quit Day

1. **Throw out your cigarettes, matches, lighters, and ashtrays the night before your quit day.** It's pretty obvious, but the less you are looking at these tempting items, the less you will think about your automatic triggers to smoke.

2. **Write down on a piece of paper the things you dislike most about smoking, and carry this paper with you as a reminder if you hit a rough patch.** Pull the paper out and read it when things get tough. It's a simple tool that can really get you through some difficult times those first few days and weeks.

3. **Switch to a brand of cigarettes you hate, or try substituting a cigar for your cigarettes (if you find cigars unpleasant) before quitting.** Again, we're looking for ways to decouple the rote act of smoking from the pleasure you think you're getting. If you're not getting pleasure from smoking, that makes it just a little easier to stop that mindless action.

4. **Declare more places in your life smoke-free so that smoking becomes more of a hassle.** Make yourself go to a new place each time you smoke, someplace you don't now associate with smoking. Again, we're breaking up the routine here, making you consciously realize every puff you take and how you feel when you're taking it.

5. **Try holding the smoke longer, and think about the negative sensations associated with breathing polluted smoke.** Really feel how your lungs react to the smoke. Picture them filling up with smoke and what they look like after your years of smoking. Not a pretty picture.

6. **Find a buddy.** In psychological circles, we call this a "reporting relationship." Choose someone who is genuinely supportive or a supportive peer group like nicotine anonymous.org, or Nicotine Anonymous in person if it is available. You can also establish a reporting relationship with a trusted health care practitioner or a member of the clergy or a good friend. Think about someone who makes you comfortable, who can honestly relate to what you are going through, and who won't pass judgment if you relapse or go through a rough period. Family members can sometimes help, but avoid anyone who might decide that this is an invitation to exert control over you or change you. The important thing about a reporting relationship is that you are accountable to another warmly supportive and understanding human being or group of human beings. Frankly, with family members this can sometimes get awfully complicated, so you be the judge!

7. **Exercise.** In designing this program, I carefully reviewed what research has to say on the role of exercise in becoming tobacco-free. One thing that can really help is to replace a poor habit such as smoking with a positive, adaptive habit. Walking, in particular, has many benefits and can also help you avoid the post-quitting weight gain so many people, especially women, complain about. At least one study of women smokers found that those who literally "talk the talk and walk the walk" (i.e., add physical activity and use the buddy system) do better trying to

quit smoking than those who try to go it alone while sitting slumped on the couch.

Michael Roizen, M.D., of the Cleveland Clinic advises smokers who come to him for help to "start walking 30 minutes every day and call or e-mail your buddy every day; no excuses." He prefers, ideally, that smokers begin at least 30 days in advance of the quit date. He also advises, "If you miss a day, reset the date and start the 30 days of never missing a walking day again." For Smoke-Free in 30 Days, we recommend that you start walking 30 minutes every day for 1 week, if possible, before your quit date.

Dr. Roizen reports great success with his walking plan to quit smoking. He also advises smokers to begin weight lifting on day eight after the quit date, and not to increase physical activity by more than 10 percent a week.

How to Set Your Quit Day

There is no ideal date to quit smoking. Some people put it off from New Year's Day to Valentine's Day, from spring to summer, from the Fourth of July to Thanksgiving, from birthday to birthday. Although ultimately only you can judge when the time is ripe, there are many things you can do to build your confidence and commitment to move forward. The behavioral and cognitive exercises in the Smoke-Free in 30 Days program are designed to help you overcome any reluctance to set and keep a quit day!

Beware of the "I'll quit tomorrow" syndrome. There is nothing magically better about some later time. Delaying the quit date often just reinforces and builds the vague sense of fear many smokers have about quitting. Even people who haven't had a day off from smoking for years, who have no way of knowing how they will react to quitting with this program, may harbor great fears of the quit day. In my experience, most smokers find they are surprised that the quit day is much easier than they feared, especially when they follow the daily steps outlined in the calendar in Part IV.

But at the same time, we don't want to launch you right into quitting without the proper preparation. In the 30-day program I lay out in Part IV of this book, day one is *not* the quit day. For the first several days of the program, we are actually preparing to quit, starting off with many of these healthy lifestyle suggestions that will lay a foundation for a successful smoking cessation program. According to my plan, the actual quit day is day 10 of the 30 days.

Why do I suggest that the quit day be day 10? This gives you a chance to consult with your prescriber and pick up patches or other medicines if you plan to use them as part of your effort. This gives you a chance to build up your confidence and motivation by working through all the exercises in this program designed to lead to a successful quit day. For those who continue to struggle after the quit day, the steps provided in the calendar for *after* the quit day will also make your adjustment to becoming smoke-free as easy as possible.

Some people are in a hurry to get started and want to quit right away; others want to spend more time preparing to get ready. However you decide, there are many roads to Rome. I wish you the easiest, most comfortable journey possible, given all your individual circumstances!

Part III

BECOMING SMOKE-FREE

CHAPTER 6

What Will Your Smoke-Free Life Be Like?

I have worked with many hard-core smoking addicts, and more often than not, people are pleasantly surprised by how easy day one is for them. This doesn't mean they won't have their issues—like forgetting and absently going for a cigarette, or getting stirred up by one of their smoking triggers. But it does show that many smokers have an exaggerated expectation of the horror of withdrawal. Most of the time, especially with the proper use of NRT, it's just not that bad.

Nicotine Withdrawal Symptoms

Still, as you can see below, nicotine withdrawal does consist of a wide range of feelings and symptoms, many of which can make people feel emotionally raw and may even feel like going through a mini-depression.

Depressed mood
Insomnia
Irritability, frustration, or anger
Anxiety
Difficulty concentrating
Restlessness
Decreased heart rate
Increased appetite or weight gain

These symptoms illustrate how psychologically tumultuous a time nicotine withdrawal syndrome can be, and how important it is to be prepared for the experience. For some people, learning to feel normal again without cigarettes is their biggest challenge. Remember that it takes time to get through tobacco withdrawal.

According to *DSM-IV*, the manual of the American Psychiatric Association:* "Withdrawal symptoms can begin within a few hours of cessation, typically peak in 1–4 days, and last for 3–4 weeks. Depressive symptoms" (after becoming smoke-free) "may be associated with a relapse to smoking."

Most people feel better over time, despite having their ups and downs; but if you feel worse depression and withdrawal over time, we strongly recommend contacting an appropriate health care professional. This will best help you safeguard your efforts to become smoke-free.

Cravings and What to Expect

Over time, cravings usually become further apart and less strong. They may spike, though, if you are experiencing one of your usual triggers, such as being upset, or if there is

---

* *DSM-IV* (Washington, DC: APA, 1994), p. 246.

someone smoking nearby. Sometimes cravings go up for no apparent reason.

Usually around 3 weeks after a smoker quits, cravings start to feel more like thoughts about smoking. Thoughts about smoking aren't as urgent or pressured as cravings. Thoughts also don't usually provoke as much anxiety or concern as cravings. If your cravings don't let up, and you are using NRT, you may need to double-check your dose.

Remember that each cigarette has approximately 1 mg of nicotine, so make sure you plan your NRT accordingly. If you're a pack-a-day smoker, you need to get 20-mg worth of nicotine per day when you first start. Don't be in a hurry to taper off. You can taper off later, as you become comfortable and confident.

If you elected not to use NRT, and your cravings persist, this may be a good time to reconsider NRT. Some people experience prolonged withdrawal, which is defined as cravings getting worse, not better, over time and especially after 5 weeks of being smoke-free. If this happens, consult a specialist.

Symptoms of, and Solutions for, Nicotine Withdrawal and Cravings

If you've ever tried and failed to quit before, these symptoms will come as no surprise to you. But the physical and emotional effects of nicotine withdrawal can be surprisingly severe. Below, you'll find some ideas about how to address some of the more common issues ex-smokers face during their initial weeks of living smoke-free.

(1) DEPRESSED MOOD

Even though you should be feeling great about quitting, it's not unusual for nicotine withdrawal to lead to feelings of depression. These feelings can sometimes be intense. Here are a few tips to keep in mind if you are suffering from a case of the blues after your quit. It's important to address this symptom since, if it persists and is left untreated, depression can trigger you to begin smoking again (among other unsavory side effects).

- Call a trusted friend who usually cheers you up.
- Write in your journal.
- Consider professional help.

(2) INSOMNIA

Lack of sleep and depression go hand in hand. Insomnia is another important symptom of nicotine withdrawal that you need to address right away to keep yourself healthy and your resolution on track. Try a few of these behaviors to help keep your slumber patterns consistent.

- Do breathing and relaxation exercises for 20 minutes before going to bed.
- Avoid caffeine after noon.
- Exercise daily.

(3) IRRITABILITY, FRUSTRATION, OR ANGER

No, it's not your imagination—nicotine withdrawal really does make you a little quicker to lose your cool. If you find yourself with a hair-trigger temper during your first smoke-free week, don't despair. These symptoms usually abate, and in the meantime try a few of these techniques.

- If your anger is directed at a specific person, write that person a letter. Decide later if it makes sense to send the letter. Sometimes just writing it is therapeutic!
- Do breathing and relaxation exercises.
- Count to 10, or take a walk to calm yourself.
- Engage in an enjoyable activity that is incompatible with being angry, such as watching a funny movie.

(4) ANXIETY

When you're stressed, your old instinct was to grab a smoke. That cue-and-response automatic relationship has to change. Here are a few specific behaviors so you can start to substitute healthy habits for a negative one.

- Do breathing and relaxation exercises.
- Play some of your favorite calming music.
- Say the "serenity prayer" and remember that this too shall pass.
- Call a positive and helpful friend for support.
- Do some self-hypnosis (see page 158).

(5) DIFFICULTY CONCENTRATING

You may feel you're "in a fog" as your body detoxifies from smoking. Do not be reluctant to take it easy on yourself during your first smoke-free week. Give your mind and your body the time and priority they need to recover.

- Make a to-do list.
- Limit or decrease your commitments.

(6) RESTLESSNESS

Once your go-to cigarette is out of the picture, you may not know what to do with yourself or your hands. It's normal to feel a bit jumpy or restless during the initial quit period. Moving your body is a good way to address these symptoms. Take stock of your body in other ways and consciously notice your movements, large and small.

- Go out for daily walking.
- Continue daily deep-slow breathing and relaxation exercises.
- Stretch your arms and legs.

(7) DECREASED HEART RATE

Some of the physical symptoms of nicotine withdrawal can be alarming. If you experience dizziness, fainting spells, shortness of breath, and chest discomfort, call a doctor.

(8) INCREASED APPETITE OR WEIGHT GAIN

It's only natural to want to replace that cigarette with a doughnut. But the physical sensation of hunger is also a very real symptom of nicotine withdrawal. Don't be too worried about your weight at the beginning of your quitting period, but do try to address this with some basic behaviors that promote wellness.

- Avoid excess sugar and starches.
- Chew nicotine gum.
- Eat low-calorie snacks such as cut-up vegetables.

- Drink some water.
- Exercise in a new way.

(9) CRAVINGS

No matter how carefully you plan, it's normal to have some cravings for a cigarette as you're breaking free from smoking. You can be prepared for this. Be conscious of how your body feels and what actions you are taking to ride this out.

- Time the craving.
- Distract yourself with reading, music, or taking a walk.
- Try chewing a cinnamon stick.
- Read over or remember your reasons for quitting.

(10) FEELING LONELY

For many people, smoking is not only a physical behavior— it's also a social one. Don't be surprised if you find yourself facing some tough emotions during your initial week of smoke-free living.

- Join a self-help group in person or online.
- Call a friend.
- Spend time with a pet or a child!
- Volunteer.

(11) COUGHING

Smoking tobacco has coated your lungs in sticky tar. The good news is that as it begins leaving your body, your lungs will feel so much better. But the bad news is that in the short term, your smoker's cough will continue—and it may even get worse as your lungs clear up. Here are a few ideas to help alleviate some of these painful physical symptoms.

- Try a hot drink like tea with honey.
- Try sugarless cough drops.
- Call a doctor if your cough persists.

(12) CONSTIPATION

Nicotine is a drug, after all, and you are in withdrawal from smoking it. Be sure to eat and drink properly to promote good overall health as your body detoxifies itself.

- Try over-the-counter remedies.
- Increase the fiber in your diet.
- Drink plenty of water.
- Call a doctor if your constipation persists.

(13) HEADACHES

Take care of yourself, and treat your body right.

- Try over-the-counter remedies.
- Try a cold pack on your neck or forehead.
- Get a massage.
- Alternate heat and cold on your neck and forehead.
- Get some fresh air.
- Call a doctor if your headaches persist.

Learning to Avoid the
Bermuda Triangle of Relapse

In addition to nicotine withdrawal symptoms, there are three triggers that many smokers commonly encounter: other smokers, alcohol, and bad moods. I call this trio the "Bermuda Triangle of relapse." The Bermuda Triangle of relapse is a place where many smokers who are doing well smoke-free get lost.

You're likely to find yourself facing some or all of the three most common high-risk situations for the would-be ex-smoker: other smokers, alcohol, and bad moods. Remember that although you may be able to cope with *one* of these high-risk situations without smoking, *two* of them at a time, such as going out drinking with some smokers, will greatly increase your odds of smoking. If all *three* of these risk factors are present—for example, going out drinking with smokers when you are in a bad mood—you are looking for trouble, and when we look for trouble we often find it. As one patient of mine used to love to say, "If you fail to plan, you plan to fail!" The following stories illustrate how alcohol, depression, and smoking, as well as being around

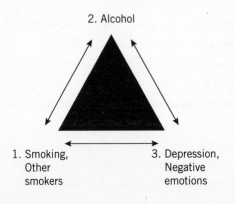

2. Alcohol

1. Smoking,
Other
smokers

3. Depression,
Negative
emotions

other people who are smoking, interact in a treacherous way to bring about relapse.

COPING WITH OTHER SMOKERS DURING WEEK ONE

Barbara S. came to her session with an important clue about her ongoing problem. Her brother with lung cancer was now living with her, and daily visitors in her apartment were smoking when they came to visit.

She had begun to smoke one or two cigarettes at night after the visitors left. Her house smelled of tobacco smoke, which triggered her cravings. Even through her brothers would go outside to smoke, they would leave the door to the outside open, and the smoke would drift in, also making her cravings worse. In the evening when she was alone, her upset over her brother and her own physical discomfort from her medical problems became "unbearable." The cigarette now became a habit and a reward for getting through the day.

She continued to smoke one to three cigarettes a day for several weeks, and felt obsessed with smoking. She now rarely used the nicotine inhaler, which had been so helpful before in getting smoke-free.

I recommended that she discuss with her brothers the problem of them smoking by the door, leaving it open, and leaving their cigarettes around her house. I also suggested that she ask her brothers to come in for a session at the clinic.

Two weeks later, she returned to the clinic 8 days smoke-free! However, she was suffering from powerful cravings. Her attitude was good, but she was struggling. When anxious, she experienced more cravings and used more nicotine cartridges. She took several puffs from one of her brother's cigarette one day, but was able to quickly reestablish her nonsmoking pattern. Her brother was getting sicker from his lung cancer, and this increased her determination, even though she felt "very, very depressed" about it.

THE ONE BUT NOT TWO RULE

Jane B. was a single patient of mine in her thirties who liked to go out to bars to socialize with her friends (this was before bars in New York City went smoke-free). She could have one drink, enjoy herself, and do all right with her friends, some of whom were still smokers and would occasionally light up. One night, however, she took a second drink of alcohol and, bingo, before she knew it, there was a cigarette in her hand and she was smoking it. She told the story to me later as if she had been in a hypnotic trance state when this happened! She realized that she could cope with one drink, but not two, so having only one drink became her rule when she was spending time with smokers.

How many drinks can you handle without smoking?

COPING WITH GETTING UPSET DURING WEEK ONE

Nathalie D., who had attended many smoking cessation programs, made the following observation: "I could always tell who would quit in the room by how angry they were. The angry ones just don't quit." Only later did I realize she was also describing herself!

Although initially she was very reluctant to share "secrets," she eventually opened up about her own life traumas. She had grown up in an orphanage, where she felt yelled at, rejected, and misunderstood. When newly smoke-free, she would go home to her husband and immediately become disappointed and angry with him. He wasn't interested in her; he was too critical of her; he didn't love her enough. Each time she came home from a different smoking cessation program, it triggered her anger, a feeling of being "less than" others. She felt overwhelmed by negative emotions and relapsed back into smoking.

According to recent research, early emotional shock and trauma are associated with an increased risk of smoking. In this case, and others I have worked with, the power of early trauma, and its damaging consequences to present-day relationships, also played a role in smoking relapse.

As Nathalie made peace with her traumatic past, she was more able to see the good things in her present. Her view of her husband changed from negative to feeling that he was a stable support and a caring person. And any negative emotions triggered by daily life with her husband stopped being a risk for relapse. We stayed in contact over many years, and she never returned to smoking.

Although Nathalie suffered through a traumatic childhood worse than most, her story illustrates a challenge many smokers share: they have to interrupt the automatic response of reaching for a cigarette when upset. When it comes to current life problems, most smokers readily see that smoking doesn't, and can't, help them cope with a real-life problem, but past hurts can be harder to disconnect from the urge to smoke.

It is not necessary to resolve the pain of an unhappy childhood or other trauma to quit smoking, but if you are in this situation, you need to understand how you have used smoking to avoid, distract yourself from, or disconnect from psychic pain. Working with a mental health professional can help, especially as quitting smoking can sometimes reveal a deep wound that needs healing.

Using Your New Awareness of Triggers as a Coping Tool

There are so many times in life when we go through the motions, repeating a behavior mindlessly just because that's the way we've always done things. Awareness is a tool that helps us make conscious choices: How will I handle smokers in my life? How will I limit or not use alcohol so I can go smoke-free? How will I cope with my irritability or nervous anxiety without mindlessly reaching for a cigarette? Part of the motivation to go smoke-free is to get back to a sense of control that the addiction to smoking prevents.

Using awareness as a tool expands the whole realm of personal control, because you are developing a life of conscious choices, a life in which you are actively participating, not passively driven by habit. Remember what the ancient Greeks said: "The unexamined life is not worth living." Developing awareness of your triggers to smoke will help you build a stronger smoke-free reality over time. Later, we will explore this notion of mindfulness further and see how it can help you make a good smoke-free adjustment and be less likely to relapse into smoking in an absentminded, unaware way.

What Will Your First Smoke-Free Month Be Like?

At around 3 weeks, some smokers report that they begin to get through longer parts of the day without even thinking about smoking. It's as if they have entered a clearing in the woods, a place of peace and calm. At the same time, even as withdrawal symptoms decrease, mind games increase, and they can enter into a new and treacherous phase of quitting.

Sometimes they let down their guard and decide to take a puff or smoke a cigar or cigarillo. Sometimes they let up on their NRT, and the cravings restart or increase. So because it seems easier now, be cautious when approaching the 3-week hump.

COPING WITH OTHER SMOKERS AT 3, 4, AND 5 WEEKS AND BEYOND

Barbara S., whose brothers insisted on smoking around her, reported that her brothers had begun to criticize her for continuing to use the nicotine oral inhaler. She was tired of serving them all their meals, and having them not help her clean up afterward or help around the house. She was under chronic stress at home, and we discussed ways for her to be more assertive with her brothers. As her resentment was building, so were her cravings to smoke. One day she got depressed and took some puffs from her brother, who was smoking in front of her in the street. Subsequently, she smoked a whole cigarette. She then seesawed between smoking and quitting. She reported high stress, depression, physical pains, and anguish about her sick brother's deteriorating condition during this time.

After further discussion about how to be assertive with her brothers, she succeeded in confronting them about their selfishness.

She gradually became less passive with her brothers, in part by enlisting support from other relatives. She started to feel better, began to lose weight, and began to have enough stamina to walk around her neighborhood, She said she no longer missed cigarettes and was feeling comfortable without them. She was confident she was not going to smoke anymore. She continued to lose weight and looked and felt better.

Her depression was better as well. Over time, she reported that she was not smoking and had completely lost interest in it.

THE ROLE OF ALCOHOL AT 3, 4, AND 5 WEEKS AND BEYOND

Over time Jane B. realized she could handle a second drink if she was with nonsmokers and in a good mood. But if she had more than one risk factor—for example, alcohol and a bad mood—she was pushing her luck with even one drink. She decided to respect, and stay within, her own limits so she could hold on to the success she was having becoming smoke-free.

THE ROLE OF NEGATIVE EMOTIONS AS A TRIGGER AT 3, 4, AND 5 WEEKS AND BEYOND

Nathalie D. was doing well and was convinced she had kicked the cigarette problem. That was before she went to see her relatives for the weekend. The visit was going fine, but on Saturday night she became enraged by her brother-in-law, who had a way of saying exactly the wrong thing. She didn't respond to his offensive remarks, but left early. On her way back to her hotel she bought a pack of cigarettes and smoked them all. In my experience, anger is one of the strongest triggers that send people back to smoking even after they have been doing well for a long time.

STRATEGY

Remember: no matter how angry you get, don't throw away your success as a nonsmoker. Your brother-in-law or whoever or whatever it is just isn't worth it! Don't make others that important or give them so much power. Living well and smoke-free is your best response to any of life's outrageous slings and arrows, insults, offenses, or misfortunes.

In their most honest moments, smokers admit that deep down they may even have started a fight or used an unpleasant situation as an excuse to smoke. This sets off a vicious circle they know deep down they will regret: feel sorry for themselves, buy a pack, feel sorry for themselves, smoke them all, get re-addicted to smoking, and feel sorry about that as well. Remember to use your self-awareness to hold on to your success no matter how bumpy a ride you are taking!

CHAPTER 7

Planning to Prevent Relapse

For many people, the biggest challenge is learning *not* to turn automatically to cigarettes when they are upset. Here are some strategies that have helped others stay tobacco-free.

1. Keep your buddy's cell number and use it when you feel a craving, or as needed. Also, keep your gum, lozenges, or inhaler with you and use for cravings or as needed.
2. Stay away from people who smoke, or speak to them in an assertive way about not smoking around you. Let them know what you are trying to accomplish so that they can be supportive.
3. Stay away from alcohol, or limit your alcohol intake, if you used to drink and smoke at the same time.
4. If you are upset, try deep, slow breathing or call someone, especially someone you really want to talk to, to distract yourself, problem-solve, or get support.

5. If you follow the walking plan, the average weight loss in 30 days is 1.4 pounds. If you are concerned about gaining weight, try:

- Accepting a few pounds because being thin from smoking is associated with poor health.
- Eating more healthy foods, eating more slowly (put your fork down between bites), and learning to enjoy food more while taking your time.
- Drinking a glass of water before you start a meal, so that you will feel fuller and less hungry.
- Developing new rituals to end your meal, like taking a walk or brushing your teeth.

6. In general, distract yourself when you get a craving or an urge to smoke, or even have thoughts about smoking. Remember, these feelings and thoughts themselves won't harm you, and they usually ease over time. If they don't, consult a health professional. Also, continue walking or other exercise, not having cigarettes at home, drinking from a water bottle, and staying away from or limiting coffee if coffee was a trigger for smoking. Develop new rituals like drinking tea or water with lemon instead of coffee.

Changing Triggers over Time

As I've said, as cravings decrease, "mind games" increase. You might start remembering smoking in a "selective" or even a "romantic" way, thinking back nostalgically to old times when you were 20, as if smoking would make you 20 again. So beware of any voices in your head that tempt or cajole you to try just one. The addiction is like a parasite. It wants to reattach itself to you and live off you! So as cravings become thoughts, beware of that troublemaking voice of addiction in your head, whispering, "Why not try 'just one'? "

Sometimes a trigger might take the form of going to a place you have not been, or seeing a person you have not seen, since you went smoke-free. People, places, and things can function as triggers, and you may find yourself, unexpectedly, thinking about smoking. If your trigger is loneliness (or being home alone), when you are busy you won't think as much about smoking. But when you are less busy, you may be more lonely, and this situation can trigger thoughts about smoking.

Worries about money can be triggers. Many people experience stress when monthly bills are due. At these times they may find themselves thinking more about smoking. Another example is drinking coffee, which typically is a stronger trigger during the first week than it is later. Later on, family problems or unpleasant emotions can be more challenging triggers. The important point is that triggers can be different at different points during your quit program.

Step one in coping with changing triggers is to identify them and think about possible ways to handle them. Triggers can surprise you. You may start craving and then realize that your host has just served you coffee! Another example could be sitting in a specific chair, which sends a message to your brain that it's time to smoke. Why? Because you did that for so many years!

Thomas M. quit relatively easily but began immediately testing himself by spending time with smoking friends. At 5 weeks he was still not smoking, but he realized he had to be careful about his triggers, which were alcohol, friends who smoked, and anxiety. He was doing a good job of coping with life's ups and downs—such as annoyance and disappointments with others—without smoking. He was thinking less and less about smoking.

At 6 weeks he had a brief slip when he became depressed, but he got back on the nonsmoking wagon. Despite experiencing a range of difficult emotions, he did not smoke. He reported having an occasional cigarillo around this time, but added that it did not increase his urge for cigarettes. He also reported two near-slips when he was exposed to smokers.

At 11 weeks he slipped again, this time when he got drunk with some friends who were smoking. After this he began a pattern of on-off smoking-stopping-slipping, which was associated with overeating and drinking too much alcohol. He was uncomfortable with all the pressure he was under in his professional life and in his healthier way of life, and he wanted to "pull back" by smoking, drinking, and overeating. It took 2 months, but he turned around the pattern of compulsive smoking, drinking, and eating and reestablished his smoke-free footing.

He continued to be smoke-free and learned to adjust to a range of emotional experiences such as boredom, anxiety, defiance, and anger. At the 2-year mark, he was still not smoking, and he was more comfortable in his nonsmoking skin and in handling his challenging work life. At 3 years, he was not smoking and was adjusting well to his continued professional successes.

Mindfulness-Based Stress Reduction

Erin Olivo, Ph.D., MPH, a colleague, is at the forefront in applying ancient and time-tested practices to the stresses of living in our fast-paced, complex society. In our discussions over the years, she has emphasized that it is very important to remember we have a choice as to how we respond to stressful situations. Practicing mindfulness-based stress reduction can help us become aware of our automatic thought patterns and habits. This awareness challenges us to perceive and accept what is happening in the moment. It also helps give us more emotional distance from our stressors, so that we can respond more effectively. Acknowledging present-moment reality "as it is" is the first step toward changing our experience of reality.

This way of approaching stress is very similar to the way we approach smoking triggers in *Smoke-Free in 30 Days*. Self-awareness is one of our most important tools, as it enables us to identify smoking triggers: an uncomfortable feeling, other smokers, or drinking alcohol. In this way we learn to disconnect our stressor—the smoking trigger—from the automatic response of smoking. Having a choice opens up a world of alternative responses that are ultimately more satisfying than smoking.

As Dr. Olivo explains, we often do things automatically, without noticing what we are doing, as if we are on auto-pilot. Your thinking mind is pulled away from the present moment, and you become literally lost in your thoughts. This happens to all of us much of the time. Mindfulness-based stress management provides an opportunity to check in with ourselves and begin to notice signs of stress before it gets out of hand. Beginning to notice the moments that we used to "tune out" can offer us helpful insights into our stress: what causes it, how we react to it, and how we can better cope with it.

In this sense you interrupt the rote aspect of your smoking. You no longer smoke unthinkingly or passively. Increasing your awareness of your triggers helps you actively make choices about how you want to respond to the moments when you would have just lit up because you were on auto-pilot. Dr. Olivo offers some specific strategies for incorporating mindfulness practices into your daily life:*

- When you wake up in the morning, before getting out of bed notice your breathing. Take a few deep, comfortable breaths.
- Be aware of how your body feels as you move from lying down to sitting up, standing, and walking.
- Pay attention as you eat. Chew slowly and completely, and notice the textures and flavors of your food. Allow your body the time it needs to digest at the end of your meal before starting your next activity.
- When talking to another person, take a moment just to listen, appreciating this person's experience of the world, though it may be different from your own.
- Practice mindful walking, consciously placing your attention on each foot as it connects with and leaves the ground.
- When standing in line or waiting, use this time to feel your feet on the ground and notice how you are holding yourself.
- Be attentive when brushing your teeth, washing, or dressing.
- Bring mindfulness to each activity throughout your day.

In order to live well without tobacco, it is important to find new routines and outlets. Take an active part in finding rewarding life activities. Develop new positive and creative outlets—"healthy escapes." The greater your sense of well-

* From Erin Olivo, Ph.D., MPH, Columbia University Medical Center; used with permission.

being, the less likely it is that some negative emotion will overwhelm you and trigger old rote and automatic smoking behavior. Remember that your emotional life is like a garden. You must work on weeding out problems, cultivating living, and growing life projects. Smoking addiction tends to crop up in unweeded gardens.

Good luck with your efforts to live well outside the cigarette box!

Part IV

YOUR SMOKE-FREE 30-DAY CALENDAR

CHAPTER 8

Smoke-free in 30 Days: Day by Day

A Word of Encouragement

You've read about all the things you can do to stop smoking—permanently. Now it is time to put your own plan into action. By following the day-by-day advice in this 30-day calendar, you will be smoke-free by the end of a month.

Each day features a quotation from someone who has gone through this process, as well as strategies from people like yourself to help you continue moving forward. There is a checklist of tasks to do that will reinforce your commitment, and suggestions about how to write in your journal to keep track of your progress. Important information and advice to keep you motivated are also part of the calendar entries. I urge you to keep a daily journal. This could be a notebook where you can write down your thoughts, complete exercises, and in general reflect on your progress from being a smoker to becoming smoke-free.

You'll see that you won't actually become smoke-free

until day 10 of this plan. Take your time and lay the ground-work for the first several days. This ensures that by the time your "quit day" arrives, you'll be well prepared and ready to succeed.

In my practice, I've found that smoking cigarettes can be indicative of other negative coping mechanisms. Smoking not only can be harmful to your physical health but can prevent you from growing as a person. Lessons learned from quitting can be used in all areas of your life—for your lifetime.

Some people doubt that they are worthy of quitting. You might also find yourself feeling defensive and thinking you cannot succeed. Of course, I can't promise that you will be successful. I can only say that if you have done everything suggested in the *Smoke-Free in 30 Days* program up to now, and if you will follow the suggestions in the calendar (Part IV), your chance of success will be great. What you get out of the program will reflect what you put into it. Many people have already learned to be smoke-free by using the advice in this book. If you stick with the step-by-step *Smoke-Free in 30 Days* calendar, you could be home free.

DAY 1

Look at your appointment calendar the evening before so you will be mentally prepared for the next day.

Quote of the Day

> *"Cigarettes keep me stuck, but I'm afraid of change. If I stop long enough to look at my life, I might have to change it."*

Fear of change, of not sticking with what's familiar, keeps many people stuck. Picture yourself a few years from now.

Imagine how you will thank yourself for the efforts you make today to get unstuck from smoking.

ASSESSING YOUR MENTAL ATTITUDE

Before you can quit smoking, you need to take a good hard look at your current habits and behaviors. Smokers tend to keep their smoking behavior vague and in the shadows of their minds and lives. The following tests and exercises are designed to get you to face head-on, in the light of day, exactly what is going on with your smoking behavior and moods. This makes it much harder for you to kid yourself about being "in control" of your smoking, or about being just a "recreational smoker." It will also help you plan for any behavioral changes or medicines that can help support your commitment and determination, and make it as easy as possible to free yourself permanently from tobacco addiction.

TASKS OF THE DAY

Begin a Smoker's Diary

Your smoking diary will help you assess what you are *doing, thinking,* and *feeling* when smoking. The diary will help you identify the situations when you expect to smoke, because you often do smoke at these times. Later, it will also help you better identify the times you might be tempted to smoke. These "triggers" to smoke can be external situations—like drinking your morning coffee or sitting around after a meal— or they can be internal, such as emotions you experience, like anger or sadness. See the sample diary page below:

Cigarette #	What am I doing?	What am I thinking?	What am I feeling?
1	Drinking my morning coffee	About a meeting later	Anxious

Ask Yourself How Addicted You Really Are to Cigarettes

As you are learning to track your triggers to smoke, let's next look more closely at how addicted you are. Take the Fagerström Dependence Test and use the scoring key below.

The Fagerström Test of Nicotine Dependence

		Points
1.	How soon after you wake up do you smoke your first cigarette?	
	Within 5 min	3
	6–30 min	2
	31–60 min	1
	After 60 min	0
2.	Do you find it difficult to refrain from smoking in places where it is forbidden?	
	Yes	1
	No	0
3.	Which cigarette would you hate most to give up?	
	The first one in the morning	1
	Any other	0
4.	How many cigarettes per day do you smoke?	
	≤10	0
	11–20	1
	21–30	2
	≥31	3
5.	Do you smoke more frequently during the first hours after waking than during the rest of the day?	
	Yes	1
	No	0
6.	Do you smoke if you are so ill that you are in bed most of the day?	
	Yes	1
	No	0

Comments to different degrees of dependence

Points	% smokers	Comments
0–1	20	Very low dependence
		Few and light withdrawal symptoms
		Seldomly need help to give up
2–3	30	A big group of smokers
		A certain degree of dependence
		Difficult withdrawal symptoms can occur
		Often manage to give up by themselves
		Medicines can be of help
4–5	30	A big group of smokers
		Overaverage dependence
		Withdrawal symptoms common
		Medicines often very helpful
		Risk for smoking-related disorders is real
6–7	15	Strong dependence and withdrawal
		Likelihood to give up smoking poor
		High risk for smoking-related disorders
		Medicines important, possibly combinations
		Higher dose, longer duration may be needed
		Support treatment important
		Depression and high alcohol intake common
8–10	5	Small group with extreme dependence
		Chances to give up are very small
		Handicapping withdrawal symptoms
		Support Rx and medicines essential, preferably over long time and in high dose
		Most will have smoking-related disorders
		Anxiety, depression, pain, and alcohol dependence common

Complete the Withdrawal Checklist

Not everyone who is addicted to smoking experiences a withdrawal syndrome. Some people don't have withdrawal problems when they quit—they feel surprisingly fine. But others can experience widely varying degrees of withdrawal. Cravings to smoke can come during smoking, and even after withdrawal is over. Withdrawal is just one part of smoking addiction, and there are many different patterns of addiction. To give yourself a sense of whether you might experience withdrawal symptoms, read the checklist to help you anticipate, and be prepared to cope with, any symptoms of withdrawal.

The withdrawal checklist below is from *DSM-IV*, the *Diagnostic and Statistical Manual* of the American Psychiatric Association. It will help you better understand this element of addiction.

Answer yes or no to the questions below:

A. Daily use of nicotine for at least several weeks   YES   NO

B. Abrupt cessation of nicotine use, or reduction in the amount of nicotine used, followed within 24 hours by four (or more) of the following signs:

    (1) Dysphoric or depressed mood   YES   NO

    (2) Insomnia   YES   NO

    (3) Irritability, frustration, or anger   YES   NO

    (4) Anxiety   YES   NO

    (5) Difficulty concentrating   YES   NO

    (6) Restlessness   YES   NO

    (7) Decreased heart rate   YES   NO

    (8) Increased appetite or weight gain   YES   NO

If you answered yes to A (smoke daily for at least several weeks) and yes to at least four of the symptoms in B, then you have a problem, and may even meet the psychiatric definition for nicotine withdrawal. Knowing this can help you face mixed feelings about your smoking addiction. Perhaps it is as serious as you feared. It can also help you build your commitment to change and to learning to breathe easier.

Your Mood and Going Smoke-Free
Even when you are smoking cigarettes:

A. Do you feel anxious and nervous and has this continued every
day for the last 2 weeks?   YES   NO

If yes, you may have more anxiety about getting through your quit day (the day you go completely tobacco-free). In that case, you may need to pay extra attention to working on preparation, confidence-building, and motivation.

B. Do you feel sad and blue and has this continued every day for
the last 2 weeks?   YES   NO

If yes, you may have more emotional discomfort after getting through the day you go completely tobacco-free. In that case, you may need to pay extra attention to planning your day-one experience to get that extra confidence that you can succeed. You may also need to carefully review coping with nicotine withdrawal symptoms, using successful strategies, and learning to live well without tobacco (see Chapters 5, 6, 7, and 8).

If you answered either A or B with a yes, look at the self-assessments in Chapter 4. It would be a good idea to take these clinical scales for depression and anxiety and review them with your family doctor to see if you would also benefit from an assessment or treatment with a mental health specialist.

If your self-assessment shows that you have lost control of your smoking behavior, that it is no longer like having a drink just on Saturday night, then seriously consider setting your goal to be completely tobacco-free. This is the surest foundation for the vast majority of smokers.

Very few addicted smokers can learn to take smoking or leave it by choice. Chances are that if you have gotten this far in the book you are *not* one of the few recreational smokers, but in fact a smoking addict. Once you stop completely, the mental and physical healing begins immediately, and most people feel a surprising sense of well-being and empowerment. What's more, just cutting down on cigarettes often amounts to no more than waiting to smoke. This is another version of the grand battle to *control your addiction* through stress and strain.

Do you just want to keep training yourself to wait for the next smoke, and stay stuck on the endless merry-go-round of addiction and withdrawal? Or do you want to break free of smoking addiction and achieve genuine freedom?

IF I COULD SIT DOWN WITH YOU . . .

"I'm no longer enjoying smoking, but I just don't know how to stop."

One hidden and little-understood reason why many people want to quit is called getting less bang for the buck. This often happens around age 40. The smoking machinery or infrastructure is not working as well; the experience becomes overrated and is just not as good as advertised. Also, by age 40 it may finally be sinking in that you are not immortal, and there will be only one body to a customer.

DAY 2

Look at your appointment calendar the evening before so you will be mentally prepared for the next calendar day.

Quote of the Day

> *"Cigarettes are my fuel to do too much. Then when I get overworked, I use them to calm down."*

HONING YOUR MENTAL ATTITUDE

Most people report that they naturally have more energy when they stop puffing smoke and start pumping more oxygen into their bloodstream. Taking deep, slow breaths as an alternative to smoking uses the body's own responses to calm and relax yourself. Surprisingly, many people feel calmer just getting off the merry-go-round of addiction, which creates its own anxiety and nervous tension.

TASKS FOR THE DAY

Fill in Your Smoking Diary for Today
See page 115.

Review
Review "How to Set Your Quit Day. See pages 82–83.

Get in Touch with Your Health Care Professional
about Smoking Cessation Medication
First, read through the options in the instructions for smoking cessation medications below, and consider which one,

if any, of these medications appeals to you most. If, after reading Chapter 4, you have decided to work with a doctor, make an appointment with your health care provider and fax him or her the form below: "Specific Instructions for Smoking Cessation Medications to Review with Your M.D., Dentist, or Nurse Practitioner." This will help you have the best possible conversation with your health care provider.

Specific Instructions for Smoking Cessation Medications to Review with Your M.D., Dentist, or Nurse Practitioner:

1. Review reasons for quitting: _____. (Frame these reasons in personal and positive ways. For example: to look and feel younger; to have more energy, better skin and fewer wrinkles, and a better sex life; etc. Try to emphasize the top three reasons.)

2. Review choice of buddy: _____. (Frame this as a chance to gain commitment from the buddy, and agree to be a buddy after you yourself have succeeded). Phone number and e-mail address for buddy: _____.

3. Walk daily for 30 minutes. The 30 minutes do not have to be a single session. Indicate, in your Tobacco-Free Plan Checklist, the date you begin your walking plan. According to Dr. Roizen: "Those that skipped a day have much higher nonsuccess rates. I have never had an ambulatory patient not able to do 30 minutes."

4. Certain forms of nicotine replacement therapy (NRT), such as patches and gum, are available without prescription at your local pharmacy. However, some insurance plans (including Medicaid) will cover NRT like the patch and the gum, so check with your plan to see if a prescription can lower your costs. You can also talk to your doctor about other medication options to make going tobacco-free as easy as possible. Below is information for you to review

with your prescriber on common medication strategies. In brief, these are: (1) nicotine patch; (2) nicotine gum; (3) nicotine oral inhaler; (4) bupropion (Zyban, Wellbutrin) alone; (5) bupropion (Zyban, Wellbutrin) plus NRT (patch, gum, or inhaler); and (6) Chantix.

5. Fill your prescriptions (your doctor will send you prescriptions).

6. You can buy a nicotine transdermal patch system at your drugstore without a prescription. (However, as noted above, some insurance plans will cover the patches by prescription only, so this is worth checking.) The 21-mg patches replace approximately a pack a day; 14-mg or 7-mg patches replace about 10 or fewer cigarettes a day. Count 1 mg per cigarette to determine which patch you should buy. When you get to your quit day, you will place the patch on your upper body (above your waist). Most people put it on a hairless part of the upper arm. You will rotate the patch daily (this helps avoid rashes). If you feel that the patch disturbs your sleep, take it off just before going to bed. Taper down to 14 mg or 7 mg as you feel successful and confident. Discuss potential side effects with your doctor (a rash is most common).

7. You can buy nicotine gum (4 mg or 2 mg) at your drugstore without a prescription. (However, as noted above, some insurance plans will cover the gum by prescription only, so this is worth checking.) Count 1 mg per cigarette to determine which gum you should buy. If you are a heavy smoker (a pack a day or more) you will definitely want the strong stuff (4-mg gum). With each piece of 2-mg gum, you absorb approximately 1 mg of nicotine, the amount found in one cigarette. With each piece of 4-mg gum, you absorb approximately 2 mg of nicotine, the amount found in 2 cigarettes. Do *not* chew nicotine gum like regular gum. Chew it a few times until there is a pep-

pery taste (which means the nicotine is being released). Then stop chewing and "park" it between your cheek and your gum. Regular use is more effective than using it just as you need it, but both are helpful. Taper the gum off as you feel more successful and confident over 2 to 3 months. Acidic beverages (coffee, tea, citrus juices, sodas) inactivate nicotine being released in the mouth, so avoid them for 15 minutes before and at time of using the gum. Discuss potential side effects with your doctor. (Nausea is common and is usually due to incorrect chewing. If you experience nausea, review chewing and "parking," above.)

8. Nicotine oral inhaler (available by prescription only). The inhaler is a thin plastic tube, which pulls apart to make room for nicotine-filled cartridges. One advantage is that when you get the urge to smoke, you can puff on the inhaler, and thus experience the ritual hand-to-mouth feel of a cigarette. Each cartridge is labeled as having 10 mg of nicotine but delivers only 4 mg, and the person absorbs approximately only 2 mg per cartridge. This means that a pack-a-day smoker needs to use approximately 10 cartridges a day. Each cartridge offers 80 puffs over 20 to 30 minutes. So 10 cartridges add up to about 800 puffs per day, enough to keep even a heavy smoker busy and distracted. Frequent puffing gives the best results. Acidic beverages (coffee, tea, citrus juices, sodas) inactivate nicotine being released in the mouth, so avoid them for 15 minutes before and at time of using the inhaler. Taper off as you feel successful and confident over 2 to 3 months. Recommended use is up to 6 months. Cold air can decrease nicotine delivery. Discuss potential side effects with your doctor. (Mouth and throat irritation and coughing are usually mild. It's best to puff gently at first.)

9. Bupropion (Zyban, Wellbutrin) is available by prescription only. The best dose of bupropion for smoking cessation is

300 mg/day. Plan to start taking bupropion 7 to 10 days before you intend to stop smoking. It can be good to start with 100-mg or 150-mg tablets and then increase to 300-mg tablets. If you use 150-mg tablets, these must be taken 8 hours apart (often, 10 AM and 6 PM are good times). Bupropion can be combined with NRT to good effect. For example: 21-mg patches replace approximately a pack a day; 14-mg or 7-mg patches replace about 10 or fewer cigarettes a day. See above for other NRT options (gum and inhaler). Take buproprion as directed by your doctor. The American Cancer Society states: "This drug should not be taken if you have ever had seizures, heavy alcohol use, serious head injury, bipolar (manic-depressive) illness, anorexia or bulimia (eating disorders)."

10. Chantix (varenicline) is available by prescription only. It should be taken with food and started 1 week prior to the target quit date. Take 0.5 mg once daily for 3 days, then 0.5 mg twice daily for 4 days. Then, starting on the target quit date, take 1 mg twice daily for 11 weeks. If you're not smoking at the end of 12 weeks, on the advice of your doctor you may continue at 1 mg twice daily for an additional 12 weeks. You may stop abruptly. There is no need to taper off. Discuss potential side effects with your doctor. (Nausea and abnormal dreams are common. It is not known if Chantix can be used safely with bupropion.) See FDA Public Health Advisory on Chantix issued on February 1, 2008, online at: http://www.fda.gov/bbs/topics/NEWS/2008/NEW01788.html.

For a description of all the available medications and their pros and cons, see the American Cancer Society Web site: http://www.cancer.org/docroot/subsite/greatamericans/content/Help_Is_Available.asp.

WHAT I WOULD TELL YOU IF I COULD SIT DOWN WITH YOU IN PERSON . . .

"The patch didn't do it for me."

They say it is a poor craftsman who blames his tools. So don't blame the medicines available to help you stop smoking. These medicines can be great tools, but they are not meant to do all the work for you; you have to do your part as well. That's what *Smoke-Free in 30 Days* is all about. Make sure to send the instructions in day two of this calendar to your physician, dentist, or nurse practitioner—whoever is going to help you with the prescriptions—and review them together.

DAY 3

Look at your appointment calendar the evening before so you will be mentally prepared for the next calendar day.

Quote of the Day

"I believe I can't handle my anger without smoking. I see myself as Goody Two-shoes but also as a rebel without a cause."

HONING YOUR MENTAL ATTITUDE

How many times have you heard a smoker say, "I had such a short fuse when I quit, I went back to smoking"? Or a statement like this: "Someone I work with actually said she liked me better when I smoked"?

Anger and irritability are common withdrawal symptoms in the first several weeks of being smoke-free. Sometimes people are overanxious to please, or overly rebellious, and smoking is a form of withdrawal from both kinds of problems. These smokers may not believe they can express themselves well or have a genuine impact on others, or they may fear making a mess of their relationships, when they no longer have a smoke screen to hide behind. Review the section in this calendar on self-assertion (page 143) to find a realistic middle way to become genuinely self-assertive.

TASKS FOR THE DAY

Schedule Your Smoking by the Clock

1. How many cigarettes do you smoke each day?
2. How many hours are you awake each day?
3. Make a rough estimate of how many cigarettes per hour, on average, you smoke

Note: Include only hours during the day when you usually smoke! For example, some people don't smoke all day at work. So you would begin with your first cigarette after work (unless, of course, you smoke at lunch or breaks).

Make seven copies of this schedule and use it for the next 7 days. If you smoke an average of two cigarettes per hour, circle "two times an hour" for those waking hours where you typically are smoking. So if you get up at 6 AM and smoke, circle 6 AM and then 6:30 AM. The point of this exercise is not to cut down on your smoking, but to schedule it so that you smoke not when you want to but only according to the schedule. The most you can schedule is every 15 minutes. If you miss a scheduled cigarette, do not make it up.

Morning

6:00 AM	7:30 AM	9:00 AM	10:30 AM
6:15 AM	7:45 AM	9:15 AM	10:45 AM
6:30 AM	8:00 AM	9:30 AM	11:00 AM
6:45 AM	8:15 AM	9:45 AM	11:15 AM
7:00 AM	8:30 AM	10:00 AM	11:30 AM
7:15 AM	8:45 AM	10:15 AM	11:45 AM

Afternoon

12:00 NOON	1:15 PM	2:30 PM	3:45 PM
12:15 PM	1:30 PM	2:45 PM	4:00 PM
12:30 PM	1:45 PM	3:00 PM	4:15 PM
12:45 PM	2:00 PM	3:15 PM	4:30 PM
1:00 PM	2:15 PM	3:30 PM	4:45 PM

Evening

5:00 PM	6:45 PM	8:30 PM	10:15 PM
5:15 PM	7:00 PM	8:45 PM	10:30 PM
5:30 PM	7:15 PM	9:00 PM	10:45 PM
5:45 PM	7:30 PM	9:15 PM	11:00 PM
6:00 PM	7:45 PM	9:30 PM	11:15 PM
6:15 PM	8:00 PM	9:45 PM	11:30 PM
6:30 PM	8:15 PM	10:00 PM	11:45 PM

Night

12:00 MIDNIGHT	12:15 AM	12:30 AM	12:45 AM

Night owls

1:00 AM	2:15 AM	3:30 AM	4:45 AM
1:15 AM	2:30 AM	3:45 AM	5:00 AM
1:30 AM	2:45 AM	4:00 AM	5:15 AM
1:45 AM	3:00 AM	4:15 AM	5:30 AM
2:00 AM	3:15 AM	4:30 AM	5:45 AM

Consider If You Are Addicted to Smoking

In the last year, was there a day you didn't smoke at all (not even a puff)?

If yes, think about how you did it and how you then went back to smoking. Try to learn from what worked and what didn't. If no—if you haven't had a day without smoking in the last year, or for many years—don't despair. The movie in your head about how impossible breaking free from smoking will be is probably greatly exaggerated. Usually, especially with proper use of medicines and a good behavioral plan, reality is much better than the scary movie in your head. Remember, it is possible to break free of smoking. Some people just have to put in a higher level of effort than others. This may not seem fair, but some people have to work harder at this to feel normal afterward.

This program is designed to help make this journey as successful as possible, with the fewest unnecessary detours. Think of the program as a guide who has been on this journey before and whose job it is to help you avoid the pitfalls and dead ends along the path to success.

Do you continue to smoke despite having a medical problem caused by tobacco—like bronchitis or chronic obstructive pulmonary disease (COPD)—or other undesirable consequences?

If yes, read the next paragraph, on continued smoking despite adverse consequences.

Smokers are well aware of the medical problems associated with smoking—after all, these problems are listed on every pack they smoke. Even when told that a problem is a matter of life and death, many continue to smoke after having a heart attack or surgery for lung or oral cancer. This behavior mystifies their loved ones and leaves even the smoker bewildered. Yet this is a hallmark of addiction and distinguishes it from "bad habits," which also involve automatic behavior. The difference is that bad habits, however annoying they may be to those around us, don't cause real and serious life consequences. Other consequences from smoking might include losing out on job or dating opportunities, or upsetting relatives, or frightening one's young children.

Do you get less bang for the buck from smoking? Do you get less of an effect (pleasure or satisfaction) from the same number of cigarettes each day?

If either yes or no, answer the questions below.

1. Do you continue to smoke, even though you enjoy only 10 to 20 percent of the cigarettes you light up?
   If yes, remember that many people get sick of their addiction over time (especially after the age of 40). What was social and fun becomes rote habit and gives less pleasure than advertised. Keeping this in mind can motivate you to move forward with your program.

2. Do you still enjoy smoking most or all of the time?
   If yes, still consider the question of smoking addiction in a hardheaded way. Is this pleasure so great that it's worth the risks to health? In one survey of how guilty they feel about smoking, smokers scored an average of 7 on a scale from 1 to 10 ("extremely guilty"). Even if you still enjoy smoking, would it also be nice to shed the burden of guilt and shame you carry because of smoking? Remember: this is your body, and there is only one body for each customer. So even with all the new replacement parts available, you still can't protect your body from all the pollution in cigarette smoke. Getting smoke-free is like taking out a new health insurance policy, but with no monthly payments!

WHAT I WOULD TELL YOU IF I COULD SIT DOWN WITH YOU IN PERSON . . .

"I try to smoke only when I drink, and with friends, but I have noticed there are times now that I have begun to smoke when no one is around."

The wish of many addicted smokers is to somehow down-shift to being just recreational smokers. Unfortunately, it usually works the other way around! Historically, only about 10 percent of smokers can do this—for instance, smoking only at a weekly card game. Over 90 percent of people can use alcohol that way, but it's the opposite with smokers. So even though addiction may sneak up on you over time, and you might not quite realize it, it's quite normal to be addicted if you are a smoker.

DAY 4

Look at your appointment calendar the evening before so you will be mentally prepared for the next calendar day.

Quote of the Day

"I used to smoke four to five packs a day. Now I smoke less than a pack and enjoy only one cigarette a day. I live with stress and conflict, and I light up when I'm stressed or in conflict. I know this doesn't make sense, because I quit once for 6 years and I was OK."

HONING YOUR MENTAL ATTITUDE

Try to be honest about what is a reason and what is an excuse to smoke. *Webster's* defines *reason* as "a good cause . . . a rational ground or motive." In contrast, an *excuse* is defined as an attempt to "remove blame," to "forgive entirely or overlook," to pardon or justify. An example of an excuse is "He was always ready to excuse himself from any responsibility for the results of his behavior." A large part of recovery from any addiction is being able to look honestly at one's behavior and tell the difference between a reason and an excuse.

TASKS FOR THE DAY

Read
Read Chapter 2 and determine what type of smoker you are.

Smoking by the Clock
Continue with this.

Think about the Most Common Reasons for Quitting
Make a note of those that apply to you—why do you want to quit smoking? To:

1. Improve my health
2. Improve the smell in my house or on my clothes
3. Protect the health of those affected by my smoking, including family members, children, and pets
4. Set a good example to others about smoking
5. Feel less shame or guilt about what I am doing
6. Increase my capacity to exercise
7. Breathe better or cough less
8. Save money on the cost of cigarettes
9. Save on the cost of illness (and lost work) from smoking
10. Make my children, who don't like it, happy

11. Make myself and my family proud
12. Feel and look younger
13. Improve my sex life, or get more dates, or both
14. Have more energy
15. Have better skin, and fewer wrinkles

DAY 5

Look at your appointment calendar the evening before day five so you will be mentally prepared for the next calendar day.

Quote of the Day

> *"I thought I would be dead at 55, so I smoked. Now I'm 56 and it looks as though I may be around for a while."*

HONING YOUR MENTAL ATTITUDE

They say it's not how you die but how you live that counts, and how well you live. Nonsmokers enjoy more independence as they age. This means less disability and fewer trips to doctors' offices.

TASKS FOR THE DAY

Smoking by the Clock
Continue with this.

Review
Review "Isn't It Safe to Smoke Just a Few a Day?" on page 5.

BUILDING YOUR POSITIVE MOTIVATIONS FOR CHANGE

To crystallize the benefits of quitting, many patients report not only that they breathe better, but they sleep better, and have more energy. Many also report less worry about getting sick when they are living tobacco-free. Even better, the benefits can extend beyond physical health to an improved sense of emotional well-being

List in your journal your positive motivations for getting started on the *Smoke-Free in 30 Days* program.

PSYCHOLOGICAL BENEFITS OF QUITTING

- Cigarette smokers are four times as likely as nonsmokers to report feeling unrested after a night's sleep.
- Smokers spend less time in deep sleep and more time in light sleep than nonsmokers. Smokers may experience nicotine withdrawal each night, and this withdrawal may contribute to disturbances in sleep.*
- A good night's rest can regulate your mood and help you cope with the next day's emotional challenges; sleep deprivation does the opposite by excessively boosting the part of the brain most closely connected to depression, anxiety, and other psychiatric disorders. Sleep disruption is present in almost all psychiatric disorders.**
- Less guilt.
- Less worry about getting sick when living tobacco-free.

GET YOUR BLOOD FLOWING

One of the participants in a group I once led could tell immediately from looking around the room who was smoking and who wasn't. All she did was notice healthy versus sallow-grayish skin on people's faces. The same improvements in the body's blood flow that bring life back to the skin may also bring more arousal and better erections in men, and easier orgasms and more sensitivity for women. Although this hasn't been proved beyond the shadow of a doubt, some research has found that nonsmokers as a group are more attractive to the opposite sex. This means that by becoming a nonsmoker you will increase the odds of having an improved sex life.

Better circulation can also give you more energy for walking, running, and other exercise. As the oxygen in your system increases, you may also experience less fatigue and fewer headaches (yes, smoking also causes headaches).

Source: *Lin Zhung et al., Power Spectral Analysis of EEG Activity during Sleep in Cigarette Smokers. *Chest*, 133, 2 (February 2008): 427–432.

** From Seung-Schik Yoo et al., "The Human Emotional Brain without Sleep—a Prefrontal Amygdala Disconnect," *Current Biology*, 17, 20 (October 23, 2007).

DAY 6

Look at your appointment calendar the evening before day six so you will be mentally prepared for the next calendar day.

Quote of the Day

"I have many worries; I get overwhelmed and turn to cigarettes for comfort and support. But they bring me no pleasure."

HONING YOUR MENTAL ATTITUDE

Most people think of the health and medical consequences of smoking, but they do not consider the emotional consequences of relying on cigarettes for comfort and support.

This becomes a knee-jerk, automatic response and a way of handling life's worries. Some smokers tell me that their friends confide in them, but they don't confide in their friends; when they are upset they turn to smoking as a "friend" instead. How can toxic smoke provide the human comfort and support of a loving friend?

TASKS FOR THE DAY

Smoking by the Clock
Continue with this.

Mental Exercise: Life Will Be Better without Smoking, Because . . .
Many people confuse breaking free of smoking with waiting to smoke. They are not the same thing! Allowing yourself to heal from smoking addiction, both mentally and physically, involves a release: letting yourself off the hook of addiction. This is a different mental approach from "hard-knuckle" willpower and toughing it out.

The "willpower only" approach can build up tension over time and set you up for a smoking relapse. How long can you hold on to the edge of a cliff? As you feel heavier over time, chances are that you will fall of your own weight. The approach I am suggesting involves releasing yourself from the addiction altogether. In this approach, the goal is accepting that life will be better without tobacco. This acceptance is emotional, not just in your surface, everyday consciousness. In other words, it takes place somewhere deep inside. Write down reasons life will be better without smoking:

_____.

So remember that you are *accepting* life without tobacco, *not* just waiting to smoke or toughing it out. But how do you make sure life without tobacco will be better? That's what this program is all about.

Start by working through the following behavioral exercises. People often find that they hold on to certain behaviors, like smoking, because they fear change or fear something strange or unfamiliar. Once they get going, however, and see the benefits of trying things in new ways, they often get excited about moving in a new direction, especially as their confidence builds that they will be successful.

Below is a list of some common trigger situations. Write down new ways to cope with them without smoking for *after you quit smoking*. The first three are filled in so you get the idea.

Common Trigger	Develop Your Personal Coping Response
Being around smokers:	1. Ask them not to smoke around you.
	2. Avoid alcohol.
	3. Wear patch or use gum as needed.
Drinking alcohol:	1. Avoid or limit alcohol for the first several weeks or until nonsmoking is established.
	2. Avoid smokers when you are using alcohol.
	3. If craving, use deep breathing to relax.
Feeling depressed, anxious, nervous:	1. Remember, it's OK to be upset—you don't need to "fix" it.
	2. Do breathing and relaxation exercises.
	3. Drink water or listen to music.
	4. Call a supportive friend.

Common Trigger	Develop Your Personal Coping Response
Drinking coffee	
After meals	
Being alone or feeling lonely	
Everyday frustrations and upsets	
Interpersonal and family problems	
Using the bathroom	
Watching TV or talking on the telephone	
When I first get up in the morning	
Weight concerns	

WHAT I WOULD TELL YOU IF I COULD SIT DOWN WITH YOU IN PERSON . . .

"What if I quit smoking and start doing something even worse to deal with my stress, like gambling?"

When it comes to quitting smoking I have a hard sell: I need to convince people it is OK to feel bad. In reality, sometimes, as when you have a loss or a setback, there may be something wrong with you if you don't feel bad. Part of the change that some people need to learn to make is to *let* themselves feel bad, and not react to pain by smoking or any other compulsive or unhealthy behavior. The bad feeling will pass; but if you smoke to smother it, you can get stuck right back at square one.

DAY 7

Look at your appointment calendar the evening before day seven so you will be mentally prepared for the next calendar day.

Quote of the Day

> *"I have a wish to be perfect. Smoking is a rebellion against this wish."*

HONING YOUR MENTAL ATTITUDE

We all have to accept certain limits in our lives, as well as imperfections in ourselves and those we love. Instead of insisting on perfection, remember: "The perfect is the enemy of the good." Don't give up on making your life better, but try focusing on what's "good enough" so you don't lose track of, or spoil, what's right in your life.

TASKS FOR THE DAY

Smoking by the Clock
Continue with this.

Journal
Write in your journal your reasons to live smoke-free versus your reasons to continue to smoke.

- What is the balance between the two sides?
- How can you build your reasons to commit to living smoke-free?
- What will be better in your life?

Read and Consider

A false belief: "I need cigarettes because I am stressed."

Here is a false belief that many smokers share: "I need cigarettes because I am stressed. I need smoking to cope with stress." You may really believe this and, like so many smokers, you use this reasoning to explain your smoking to yourself. But what if it's just a belief, not a fact? What if smoking is just an overrated activity, a bad habit, a rote negative behavior having nothing to do with stress management? Perhaps it distracts you when you're upset. But can smoking solve real-life problems? No—it *is* a real-life problem.

This is the classic false belief of addicted smokers, and it must be challenged and debunked so you can learn to live smoke-free. When did smoking a cigarette ever solve a real-life problem? Smoking because of stress is called a rationalization. This is what you tell yourself to try to make yourself feel good about something you really feel bad about. We all engage in rationalizations of one sort or another, and smokers are especially prone to rationalize about stress and smoking.

The truth about stress and smoking: an addicted smoker doesn't need a reason to smoke.

The momentum of smoking, its automatic quality, is a three-headed monster. It comes from:

1. The effect that smoking cigarettes has on your brain and body
2. The repetitive, habitual nature of smoking
3. The role of the smoker's social environment, primarily exposure to other smokers and smoke, which are contagious

The truth: Smoking is an uncreative, repetitive response to life stress. It actually weakens the opportunity to develop healthy, flexible coping responses, because the smoker relies on a fixed, rote way of responding to the ups and downs of life.

Are you clear and confident in your commitment to changing?

Find Support

This could be professional support, or you can look among your smoking friends for peer support. A supportive peer might be someone who is also addicted to smoking and is seriously facing the same kinds of challenges as you. Another place to look for support is among peers who have already addressed their smoking addiction; still another is a self-help group like Nicotine Anonymous (Nicotine Anonymous World Services, 419 Main Street, PMB #370, Huntington Beach, CA 92648. Phone: (415) 750-0328). Nicotine Anonymous has online groups available at: http://www.nicotine-anonymous .org/.)

A health professional, therapist, or doctor who has training with smoking addiction can also be a great source of support and can help counsel you on making positive life changes to support your decision to be tobacco-free. Prescribers—medical doctors, dentists, or nurse practitioners—can also help you choose and properly use medications available to help you meet your goal. (See Chapter 4, "Do You Need a Doctor to Quit?")

WHAT I WOULD TELL YOU IF I COULD SIT DOWN WITH YOU IN PERSON . . .

"I realize my mental attitude must change. I see friends quit and I am disappointed with myself. I feel very, very guilty and keep reminding myself that other people can stop and I can't. I feel bad but don't do what will make me feel better. Today I didn't smoke, and I feel better already."

It's common to see people beating themselves up and putting themselves down over their smoking addiction. This can become just another reason to smoke, because you feel so bad. Or it can become a distraction from the real work of making changes. Often smokers just keep repeating to themselves and others how bad or weak they feel as they go on lighting up and smoking. So it's important to try to keep your outlook positive, and to take constructive actions.

DAY 8

Look at your appointment calendar the evening before day eight so you will be mentally prepared for the next calendar day.

Quote of the Day

"Smoking was my 'bottle courage.' It bought me time to deal with things. Now that I've stopped, I engage more. I am coping fine with my life. Strangely, I am calmer, more relaxed. I am OK with handling my own problems and I just try to stay away from normal, routine, daily problems if they are someone else's problems. I leave those to others now. I used to have cravings when I got upset, but I'm learning not to get upset."

TASKS FOR THE DAY

Smoking by the Clock
Continue with this.

Write a Paragraph in Your Journal for Each of the Questions Below
Writing about your experiences—in this case, smoking—has been shown to have an important impact on behavior change, and even on your health.

1. What about other smokers in your life—either at home, at work, or at play? How will you handle them?
2. What about alcohol? How will you be careful not to take a smoke while drinking? (Smoking while drinking happens to so many people who want to go smoke-free.)
3. What about bad moods and stress? How will you handle them without your automatic response of smoking?

Learn to Be Assertive and Effective with Other Smokers
Smoking cessation programs have always included assertiveness training so smokers can learn to deal skillfully with interpersonal problems as they adjust to living tobacco-free. Think of the old stereotype of smokers who are so irritable when they quit that people around them say, "Why don't you go back to smoking? I liked you better that way!"

Being assertive with smokers in your life means knowing what you want from them—usually, not to smoke in front of you—and telling them about it. But here's the rub. Many people who fear they won't be heard or listened to, or who aren't used to speaking up, don't come out with what they want directly. Instead, they may take the passive road and wait for someone to read their minds; this approach is not likely to succeed. Or they may try to control, coerce, attack, or (that dreaded word) "manipulate" other people to get their way. In this case, they are being dominant and aggressive, not genuinely self-assertive, and these tactics have a way of getting other people's backs up.

We recommend just coming out with what you want to say as directly and honestly as you can. Most people (even when they themselves smoke!) sincerely want to help others struggling to get free of smoking addiction. So go ahead. Ask if they can smoke outside so you won't be tempted. Ask if you can get together at a smoke-free place so you won't be tempted. This way, they will know what you want and will have a chance to respond positively. This way, they won't be failing a test they don't even know they are taking. Take a risk; be assertive. It's for a good cause: you.

WHAT I WOULD TELL YOU IF I COULD SIT DOWN WITH YOU IN PERSON . . .

"Some of my friends quit, and without much trouble. What's wrong with me?"

Not all smokers are alike, so beware of comparing apples with oranges. Some smokers quit relatively easily, and on their own. Some, as I'm sure you've heard, say quitting is the hardest thing they have ever done. Part of why quitting is so difficult for some people is that they have to discover their own best way, through trial and error. *Smoke-Free in 30 Days* is designed to give all smokers who want to quit the best available tools and guidance to make this as easy and successful as possible for them.

DAY 9

Look at your appointment calendar the evening before day nine so you will be mentally prepared for the next calendar day.

Quote of the Day

> *"Despite many frustrations, I'm not thinking I'll solve them by having a cigarette. Not smoking seems to be the one thing I have under control. It gives me a sense of achievement. I realize I can handle my life without the cigarette."*

HONING YOUR MENTAL ATTITUDE

If you are waiting to get everything in your life under control before you quit smoking, you may just be putting this off indefinitely. Not putting smoke in your body can be one thing to feel good about while you are trying to get a handle on your other problems.

TASKS FOR THE DAY

Smoking by the Clock
Continue with this.

Reading
Reread Chapter 7, "Planning to Prevent Relapse."

Checklist
Copy and complete this *Smoke-Free Plan Checklist* so you can be confident about how prepared you are to move forward:

1. Reviewed medications available to make it easier to go completely smoke-free (Chapters 3 and 4).
2. Discussed medications that interest you with your doctor, dentist, or nurse practitioner.
3. Decided to use or not use medication to help with your plan. If you decided to use NRT:
   a. Do you have or need a prescription?
   b. Do you know how to use it?
4. Decided to use other medications:
   a. Zyban:
      Do you have a prescription?
      Do you know how to use it?
   b. Chantix:
      Do you have a prescription?
      Do you know how to use it?
5. Chose a specific date to go completely smoke-free (according to our 30-day plan, that day is tomorrow).
6. Carry a water bottle.
7. Use deep, slow breathing exercises to relax, distract yourself when upset, and cope with cravings.
8. Avoid smokers.
9. Speak with nonsmokers to get them to support your efforts.
10. Make sure there are no cigarettes in your home.
11. Avoid or limit alcohol.
12. Start or continue a daily 30-minute walking program.

Relaxation Breathing

Most of us pay little or no attention to our breathing, but it provides an important clue to how we are feeling. This relaxation technique will enrich your awareness of your body and mind and help you cope better with stress and cravings as a nonsmoker. The breath can also be a very powerful and effective tool for managing stress. After completing even 10 relaxation breath cycles, you should feel calmer and more relaxed, physically and mentally.

Try this simple exercise:

- Sit upright in a comfortable chair or use pillows behind your back to provide support. Tuck in your chin slightly to provide space in the back of your neck and chest.
- Now bring your attention to your breath. You may choose to close your eyes as you do this.
- Breathe in slowly through your nose, letting your belly expand outward as you do so.
- Exhale slowly and completely, letting your belly fall inward.
- Follow the natural rhythm of your breath, concentrating on the movement of your belly as you breathe easily.
- As you do this, notice any tightness you might be holding in any area. Gently encourage your body to let go as you exhale, using the breath as a guide.*

DAY 10: THE QUIT DATE

Look at your appointment calendar this evening to antici-pate problems and develop strategies for the next calendar day. For example, will there be stress, another smoker, or a gathering with smoking or alcohol, and how do you plan to handle these triggers?

---

* From Erin Olivo, Ph.D., MPH, Columbia University Medical Center; used with permission.

Quote of the Day

> *"In the past, I took puffs (from other people's cigarettes) and the cravings never got better. This time I'm avoiding my smoking friends. My son also smokes but says he wants to be supportive and will have only one cigarette when he visits and will smoke it out the kitchen window."*

STRATEGY OF THE DAY

Learn new ways to relax. Try deep, slow breathing "stomach breathing" (see pages 146–47) for cravings and stress. Talk to yourself and tell yourself, "Smoking is not an option."

TASKS FOR THE DAY

Triggers to Watch Out For Today
Other smokers, alcohol, stress.

Chart Your Cravings
Low, medium, high.

Chart Your Mood
Fair, good, upset, very upset.

Journal
Write in your journal how you plan in advance to handle today's triggers, and how you will cope with your cravings and mood today and tomorrow, without smoking!

COPING WITH NICOTINE WITHDRAWAL SYMPTOMS, IF YOU HAVE THEM

Note the withdrawal symptoms that apply to you today:

Depressed mood

Insomia

Irritability, frustration, or anger

Anxiety

Difficulty concentrating

Restlessness

Decreased heart rate

Increased appetite or weight gain

Each cigarette has approximately 1 mg of nicotine, so make sure you plan your NRT accordingly. If you're a pack-a-day smoker, you need to get 20-mg worth of nicotine per day when you first start. Then taper off as you become comfortable not smoking.

Withdrawal and Emotional Upset: Nicotine withdrawal consists of a wide range of emotions and symptoms, many of which are similar to going through a mini-depression. These symptoms illustrate how emotional nicotine withdrawal syndrome can be. For many people this is their biggest challenge: learning to feel normal again without cigarettes.

WHAT I WOULD TELL YOU IF I COULD SIT DOWN WITH YOU IN PERSON . . .

"I cook for everyone and support my family, and I'm happy to do it. Smoking is the one thing I do just for myself."

I often hear the complaint that smoking (or drinking) is "the one thing I do which is purely selfish." Perhaps this person is too much in a caretaker role in her life. Smoking allows her to act on the idea that, "Not only do I not want to take care of anyone else anymore; I don't even want to be responsible for taking care of myself!"

Selfish is a terrible word in our culture. Addiction is an example of *unhealthy selfishness*. However, walking each day, or making sure you get to the gym several times a week, may be healthy self-interest or, in other words, *healthy selfishness*. Just as when adults on a plane are told to put oxygen masks on themselves before putting masks on their children, you have to take care of yourself first so you can be there for others when they need you. Healthy selfishness means it is possible for us to better balance our needs with the needs of others. If resentment is the royal road to smoking, perhaps when we feel more balanced between our needs and the

VISUALIZING PEACE OF MIND AND FREEDOM FROM SMOKING

1. First, picture yourself holding on to the side of a mountain. Your arms tire and your muscles ache. You are waiting to fall, waiting to let go, waiting to relapse, to smoke.

2. Now picture yourself swinging open a prison door. You are free; the wide world is open before you. You are no longer trapped, but you are nervous about making it on your own. You know that your freedom from smoking depends on maintaining an attitude of commitment or "steadfastness of purpose." Removing doubt about your choice to live smoke-free leads to peace of mind, an acceptance of living smoke-free, which can be the greatest gift of all.

needs of others there is less of a trigger to smoke—because there is less smoldering resentment at being overly selfless.

DAY 11

Look at your calendar this evening to anticipate problems and develop strategies for tomorrow. For example, will there be stress, another smoker, or a gathering with smoking or alcohol, and how do you plan to handle these triggers?

Quote of the Day, 2 Days Smoke-Free

> *"I feel better without smoking; my asthma is better; but I still believe I need to smoke to feel good. It doesn't make any sense. Smoking is my enemy, but I look forward to it. I say I don't have money, but I spend it on cigarettes; that doesn't make sense, either."*

STRATEGY OF THE DAY

It's helpful to believe that being uncomfortable now will pay off later. If you don't have the cigarette now, you can find other things to look forward to, like tasting food, being able to exercise without feeling breathless, or not having to go outdoors on a cold day to smoke.

TASKS FOR THE DAY

Triggers to Watch Out For Today
Other smokers, alcohol, stress, or other triggers.

Chart Your Cravings Today
Low, medium, high.

Chart Your Mood Today
Fair, good, upset, very upset.

Journal
Write in your journal how you plan in advance to handle today's triggers, and how you will cope with your cravings and mood today and tomorrow without smoking.

COPING WITH NICOTINE WITHDRAWAL SYMPTOMS IF YOU HAVE THEM

Note which withdrawal symptoms apply to you today.

Depressed mood
Insomnia
Irritability, frustration, or anger
Anxiety
Difficulty concentrating
Restlessness
Decreased heart rate
Increased appetite or weight gain

How will you cope? Write your strategy for today in your journal. See Chapter 6 for a list of suggested coping strategies for withdrawal symptoms.

DAY 12

Look at your appointment calendar this evening to anticipate problems and develop strategies for tomorrow. For example, will there be stress, another smoker, or a gathering with

LEARN THE BODY SCAN
MINDFULNESS EXERCISE*

The "body scan" exercise can enrich your awareness of your body and mind and help you cope better with stress and cravings. It is a simple and effective mindfulness technique (see pages 106–9). If you become distracted, you can just pick up where you drifted off. You can practice a short body scan right now.

Begin with noticing your body in your chair. Feel the weight of your body supported by the seat beneath you. Now pay attention to the natural flow of breath. **(You are not trying to change it, but simply noticing. As thoughts arise, try not to unpack them or judge them. Simply notice them and return to the breath.)** Move on to toes, feet, legs, buttocks, pelvic area, hips, belly, torso, shoulders, arms, hands, fingers, neck, scalp, face, jaw, tongue, eye sockets, and back to the breath. Slowly bring your attention back to the whole body, the room. Open your eyes slowly when you are ready.

Did you notice places in your body that were harder to scan? Any places where you carried tension that you were unaware of? Were you able to release it? Did you find yourself carried away by thoughts? Were you able to come back to the breath? Were you surprised at how frequently your attention drifted?

By practicing mindfulness and paying attention to our mind and bodies, we can begin to take more control and switch off the autopilot. Paying attention is not the answer to all of life's problems; but all of life's problems *can* be seen more clearly when our mind is clear. Awareness enables us to respond to stressful situations by making conscious choices instead of reflexive, automatic ones. Learning to be fully aware of our body sensations and our thoughts and emotions, whether they are pleasant or unpleasant, can help us deal more effectively with our stress.

* From Erin Olivo, Ph.D., MPH, Columbia University Medical Center; used with permission.

smoking or alcohol, and how do you plan to handle these triggers?

Quote of the Day

> *"I thought my cravings increased for no reason at all. There was just this little devil over my head telling me to smoke. I was thinking: if this is a test, I am going to pass the test. A friend died four months ago because of cigarettes—lung cancer destroyed him. When I get upset about it, my cravings increase. Also, I went to see some people the other day, and they gave me coffee. Before this I wasn't craving a cigarette very much. When I look back, I can usually find something that was a trigger to increase cravings."*

TASKS FOR THE DAY

Triggers to Watch Out For Today
Other smokers, alcohol, stress, other triggers.

Chart your cravings today
Low, medium, high.

Chart Your Mood Today
Good, fair, upset, very upset.

Journal
Write in your journal how you plan in advance to handle today's triggers, and how you will cope with your cravings and mood today and tomorrow without smoking.

COPING WITH NICOTINE WITHDRAWAL SYMPTOMS IF YOU HAVE THEM

Note which symptoms apply to you today.

Depressed mood
Insomnia
Irritability, frustration, or anger
Anxiety
Difficulty concentrating
Restlessness
Decreased heart rate
Increased appetite or weight gain

How will you cope? Write your strategy for today in your journal. See Chapter 6 for a list of suggested coping strategies for withdrawal symptoms.

WHAT I WOULD TELL YOU IF I COULD SIT DOWN WITH YOU IN PERSON . . .

"If I'm feeling down, I am more likely to crave cigarettes, but sometimes a craving happens for no reason. Being around smokers increases cravings. I have taken some puffs from their cigarettes just because I was around them.

"I sometimes remove myself from smokers, but it is not always possible. My brother is a smoker, and he is coming to stay with me. I remember I was successful for three months of not smoking four years ago, but I relapsed when I was around my brother.

"I had a cold at the time, so I had fewer cravings and used less of the nicotine inhaler and didn't realize I still needed it. I don't believe my brother cares whether I relapse again or not. In

fact, I think he smokes around me on purpose, so that I will fail. I know a lot of people who relapse just because they are around smokers."

Especially in the beginning, and until you are on a good track, try to avoid smokers and smoke. It is difficult to over-state how much smoke and smokers stir up the addiction once you have banished it from your daily life. The addic-tion is always looking for an opportunity to reassert its rule, and there is no better chance than when there is another smoker nearby! You can always leave a party, or move to a different room, if there is smoking around you. If you have smokers in your home, try to negotiate with them to smoke only outside or in certain areas where you won't smell the cigarettes. Reread the section on assertiveness as needed! (See page 143).

DAY 13

Look at your appointment calendar this evening to anticipate problems and develop strategies for tomorrow. For example, will there be stress, another smoker, or a gathering with smoking or alcohol, and how do you plan to handle these triggers?

Quote of the Day

"When I have a problem the cravings are even stronger, but I speak to myself and say, 'I can't and shouldn't smoke.' The most important thing is what to do with the anxiety. I'm jumpy a lot, but I keep saying, 'You can't smoke; it's not an option.' "

STRATEGY OF THE DAY

Try saying to yourself, "Smoking is not an option."

TASKS FOR THE DAY

Triggers to Watch Out For Today
Other smokers, alcohol, stress, other triggers.

Chart Your Cravings Today
Low, medium, high.

Chart Your Mood Today
Good, fair, upset, very upset.

Journal
Write in your journal how you plan in advance to handle today's triggers, and how you will cope with your cravings and mood today and tomorrow without smoking!

COPING WITH NICOTINE WITHDRAWAL SYMPTOMS IF YOU HAVE THEM

Note which withdrawal symptoms apply to you today.

Depressed mood
Insomnia
Irritability, frustration, or anger
Anxiety
Difficulty concentrating
Restlessness
Decreased heart rate
Increased appetite or weight gain

How will you cope? Write your strategy for today in your journal. See Chapter 6 for a list of suggested coping strategies for withdrawal symptoms.

TECHNIQUES FOR COPING WITH TRIGGERS FOR CRAVINGS

Try some self-hypnosis as a positive escape. Close your eyes and picture yourself in a park or at a beach. Feel the sun on your neck or the salty mist from the waves. Smell the sea air or the fresh grass. Picture the clouds rolling in the blue sky and afternoon making surprising shapes. Use your deep, slow breathing exercises to renew yourself and find a peaceful island that is all your own. When you open your eyes, remember your special place so you can visit it as often as you like as you adjust to your "new normal" life and daily routine.

Trigger Alert! Weight Gain

1. Watch sugar and alcohol intake.
2. Eat fresh food and put a lot of color, such as fruits and vegetables, on your plate.
3. Eat something for breakfast, even if just yogurt or a healthy cereal. Not eating until later in the day can set off a negative pattern, and your body may even store more fat if it thinks you are running short on food.
4. Cope with hunger pangs: prepare and have ready snacks such as cut-up raw vegetables.

Trigger Alert! After a Meal

Find a new ritual, such as getting up for a walk or brushing your teeth.

Trigger Alert! Craving

1. Time how long each craving lasts and learn to picture yourself riding or surfing a wave into the shore. By the time you reach the beach and feel the sun on your neck, the craving will have passed.
2. Use the nicotine oral inhaler, gum, or lozenge until the cravings pass.

Trigger Alert! Need for Something to Do with Your Hands

1. Try knitting, playing with a rubber band, or doing a jigsaw puzzle or crossword puzzle.
2. Use a cinnamon stick to distract yourself, and form a new hand-to-mouth routine.

Trigger Alert! Anxious Feeling

Use slow and deep breathing to relax until the urge to smoke passes. Take a shower.

Visit the "distraction department": Drink water, suck on ice chips, use sugarless gum or sugarless mints. Touch your toes. Play cards. Do stretches. Doodle. Read a good book! Take a piece of paper and calculate how much money you are saving. Plan something you can look forward to as a reward to do with your savings! Try talking to yourself and saying, "Smoking is not an option" or "I want to protect my body, which is my most precious asset!"

Think about providing a positive model for those who still smoke. Just as smoking can be contagious, so can quitting!

Trigger Alert! Other Smokers

During the first several weeks, avoid people, places, and things that remind you of smoking. If you do spend time with smokers, (1) keep moving if they light up; (2) avoid or limit alcohol; and (3) avoid any emotionally upsetting discussions or arguments, which may put you at more risk of smoking!

Trigger Alert! Feeling Sad or Blue
Call a friend; listen to music. If feeling sad or blue persists longer than usual or if you are thinking of hurting yourself, reach out to a trusted health care practitioner, or go to your local emergency room!

DAY  14

Look at your appointment calendar this evening to anticipate problems and develop strategies for tomorrow. For example, will there be stress, another smoker, or a gathering with smoking or alcohol, and how do you plan to handle these triggers?

Quote of the Day

> *"When I get nervous and the craving is increasing, I know I need to do something about it."*

STRATEGY OF THE DAY

Try to force your mind onto another subject, the way you switch channels on a TV. Before you know it, the craving will pass.

TASKS FOR THE DAY

Triggers to Watch Out For Today
Other smokers, alcohol, stress, other triggers.

Chart Your Cravings Today
Low, medium, high.

Chart Your Mood Today
Fair, good, upset, very upset.

Journal
Write in your journal how you plan in advance to handle today's triggers, and how you will cope with your cravings and mood today and tomorrow without smoking.

COPING WITH NICOTINE WITHDRAWAL SYMPTOMS IF YOU HAVE THEM

Note which withdrawal symptoms apply to you today.

  Depressed mood
  Insomnia
  Irritability, frustration, or anger
  Anxiety
  Difficulty concentrating
  Restlessness
  Decreased heart rate
  Increased appetite or weight gain

How will you cope? Write your strategy for today in your journal. See Chapter 6 for a list of suggested coping strategies for withdrawal symptoms.

DAY 15

Look at your appointment calendar this evening to anticipate problems and develop strategies for tomorrow. For example,

ALTERNATIVE THERAPIES

ACUPUNCTURE

Body and ear points are selected and stimulated through a variety of methods, including needles. This is believed to decrease withdrawal. Behavioral changes and counseling for emotional adjustment may also be required.

HYPNOSIS

Uses trance work to reduce resistance to behavior change. It can reinforce a smoker's desire for change, but cannot create this desire.

will there be stress, another smoker, or a gathering with smoking or alcohol, and how do you plan to handle these triggers?

Quote of the Day

"I'm very happy about quitting, but I gained 12 pounds. I'm positive I can lose weight when the craving is not around. I am eating more because of the cravings, but it's much better than in the beginning."

STRATEGY OF THE DAY

It is usually good advice to get past the early withdrawal phase before engaging in any strenuous changes in your diet beyond adopting healthy eating and exercise habits. After early withdrawal cravings begin to be more manageable and more like thoughts, without the rawness or pressure of real cravings, you can think about cutting down on your food intake and on sugars, fats, and other unhealthy foods that might be a particular problem.

TASKS FOR TODAY

Triggers to Watch Out For Today
Other smokers, alcohol, stress, other triggers.

Chart Your Cravings Today
Low, medium, high.

Chart Your Mood Today
Good, fair, upset, very upset.

Journal
Write in your journal how you plan in advance to handle today's triggers, and how you will cope with your cravings and mood today and tomorrow without smoking!

COPING WITH NICOTINE WITHDRAWAL SYMPTOMS IF YOU HAVE THEM

Note which withdrawal symptoms apply to you today.

Depressed mood
Insomnia
Irritability, frustration, or anger
Anxiety
Difficulty concentrating
Restlessness
Decreased heart rate
Increased appetite or weight gain

How will you cope? Write your strategy for today in your journal See Chapter 6 for a list of suggested coping strategies for withdrawal symptoms.

STRATEGIES TO COPE WITH CRAVINGS, WANTING TO EAT, AND GAINING WEIGHT

To help you keep your weight under control while quitting, choose forms of NRT such as the inhaler, gum, or lozenge that promote new daily rituals. These new rituals offer alternatives to automatic smoking or eating in response to cravings. These forms of NRT also help keep down weight in the crucial early stages of quitting, when cravings are typically most challenging. As cravings decrease and your confidence increases, you can begin to focus on new ways to increase your metabolism through exercise, and continue to build on your nonsmoking success by selecting foods, like fruit and vegetables, lean forms of protein, and whole grains, that will help you feel even better.

We know unhealthy behaviors often go together: for example, smoking and heavy drinking, or sedentary behavior and overeating. By becoming smoke-free, you can break a chain of various unhealthy behaviors. By engaging in exercise and eating good food in healthy amounts, you can continue to build on your great health achievement: becoming smoke-free.

Healthy Eating to Help Avoid Gaining Weight as You Go Smoke-Free

Pay attention to the difference between hunger, which is a feeling of emptiness in the stomach; and a nervous stomach, which develops when anxiety serves as a trigger for eating. *Hunger* is primarily a physical sensation; a *nervous stomach* is primarily emotional, with less of a physical component.

Eating for pleasure or nourishment is different from emotional eating. Eating can be a deeply enjoyable experience, and it also is necessary for maintaining life. But eating also carries a lot of emotional meaning. In many, if not most, cultures, food equals love. But it is possible to have too much of a good thing, like overwatering a plant, or overfeeding your family or customers in a restaurant. As a society, we have been increasing plate and portion sizes, but we have never changed how we show our appreciation for this kind of love: by cleaning our plate!

What does a healthy plate look like? Dr. Wahida Karmally, director of nutrition for the Irving Institute for Clinical and Translational Research and an associate research scientist at Columbia University Medical Center, is fond of saying, "Make sure more than half your plate is filled with color from fruits and vegetables." She adds that the meat on your plate should be "no bigger than the size of a woman's palm." Another thing to consider: if you go out to eat and you save half your meal for later, you can save on food costs! Consider taking doggie bags home from restaurants, for example.

When you are nervous or anxious, look for nonfood rewards such as:

- Relaxing a nervous stomach with breathing, not food
- Having a heart-to-heart talk with a friend, or writing in a journal
- Doing something creative

Healthy alternatives to overeating:

- Drink water before a meal to moderate hunger.
- Eat slowly, putting your fork down between bites.
- Rediscover the pleasure of tasting food as your taste buds come back to life.

DAY 16

Look at your appointment calendar this evening to anticipate problems and develop strategies for tomorrow. For example, will there be stress, another smoker, or a gathering with smoking or alcohol, and how do you plan to handle these triggers?

Quote of the Day

> *"Addiction is a game. It goes like this: 'Just one more with coffee.' But it is never just one more. I feel horrible guilt. I hide from my neighbors and tell my mother I'm having only a few, but it's a lie. I fear being without cigarettes. I believe I can't be without them. They give me pleasure, but they make me miserable and I don't like who I am when I smoke."*

HONING YOUR MENTAL ATTITUDE

Addiction is like a bus leaving a station: you are either on the bus or off it. No matter how much you try to prove you can control your addiction, and keep trying to smoke just a little, you can't have it both ways. The only exit strategy is to quit completely and get off the bus.

TASKS FOR THE DAY

Triggers to Watch Out For Today
Other smokers, alcohol, stress, other triggers.

Chart Your Cravings Today
Low, medium, high.

Chart Your Mood Today
Fair, good, upset, very upset.

Journal
Write in your journal how you plan in advance to handle today's triggers, and how you will cope with your cravings and mood today and tomorrow without smoking

COPING WITH NICOTINE WITHDRAWAL SYMPTOMS IF YOU HAVE THEM

Note which withdrawal symptoms apply to you today.

Depressed mood
Insomnia

SOME WARNING SIGNS ON ALCOHOL TO LOOK OUT FOR

Having five or more drinks at one time, for a man (four or more for a woman)

Having more than two drinks a day (or 14 a week) for men and more than one drink a day (or seven a week) for women.

For answers to frequently asked questions, see National Institute on Alcohol Abuse and Alcoholism at: http://www.niaaa.nih.gov/FAQs/General-English/default.htm.

If you fit these criteria, you are not alone! It is estimated that at some time in their lives about three out of 10 Americans develop risky patterns of drinking alcohol.

Irritability, frustration, or anger

Anxiety

Difficulty concentrating

Restlessness

Decreased heart rate

Increased appetite or weight gain

How will you cope? Write your strategy for today in your journal. See Chapter 6 for a list of suggested coping strategies for withdrawal symptoms.

DAY 17

Look at your appointment calendar this evening to anticipate problems and develop strategies for tomorrow. For example, will there be stress, another smoker, or a gathering with smoking or alcohol, and how do you plan to handle these triggers?

Quote of the Day

"When I get upset, I have stronger cravings. It's always been that every time I'm upset I would smoke; now I crave a cigarette more. I drink water and sometimes use deep breathing to get through it. I don't want to smoke, so even if I have cravings, that doesn't mean I will smoke."

STRATEGY OF THE DAY

Cravings are time-limited. Picture yourself on a wave and ride it in to the shore; breathe deeply to calm yourself and distract yourself. When it's over, sit on the beach and feel the sun on your neck.

TASKS FOR THE DAY

Triggers to Watch Out For Today
Other smokers, alcohol, stress, other triggers.

Chart Your Cravings Today
Low, medium, high.

Chart Your Mood Today
Good, fair, upset, very upset.

Journal
Write in your journal how you plan in advance to handle today's triggers, and how you will cope with your cravings and mood today and tomorrow without smoking!

CHARTING CRAVINGS OVER TIME

In my drawing below, the top line indicates what cravings are like if you continue to smoke. The bottom lines show how cravings decrease over time, while still spiking occasionally.

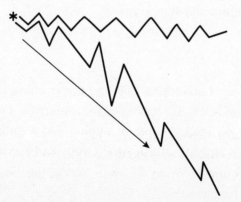

Cravings typically last between 2 to 4 and 3 to 5 weeks, and they go up and down over time. Don't be discouraged if yours go up. It's often just a temporary spike and will pass if you roll with it. You'll notice that over time, cravings get shorter, less intense, and further apart, even if you have some bad times along the way.

COPING WITH NICOTINE WITHDRAWAL SYMPTOMS IF YOU HAVE THEM

Note which symptoms you have today.

Depressed mood
Insomnia
Irritability, frustration, or anger
Anxiety
Difficulty concentrating
Restlessness
Decreased heart rate
Increased appetite or weight gain

How will you cope? Write your strategy for today in your journal. See Chapter 6 for a list of suggested coping strategies for withdrawal symptoms.

DAY 18

Look at your appointment calendar this evening to anticipate problems and develop strategies for tomorrow. For example, will there be stress, another smoker, or a gathering with smoking or alcohol, and how do you plan to handle these triggers?

Quote of the Day

"I'm having cravings sometimes, but not every day. They get worse with family problems, bad news, or family arguments. I know it's not a solution if I 'try one.' I just use water or sugar-free candy. I would feel guilty if I took 'just one.' I would be really, really killing myself to go back to that. I'm having less coffee, since I'm less interested now that I'm not smoking. I just have a little in the morning. With no coffee or cigarettes, I am sleeping much better. I'm more rested than before in the morning."

TASKS FOR THE DAY

Triggers to Watch Out For Today
Other smokers, alcohol, stress, other triggers.

Chart Your Cravings Today
Low, medium, high.

Chart Your Mood Today
Good, fair, upset, very upset.

Journal
Write in your journal how you plan in advance to handle today's triggers, and how you will cope with your cravings and mood today and tomorrow without smoking!

COPING WITH NICOTINE WITHDRAWAL SYMPTOMS IF YOU HAVE THEM

Note which symptoms you have today.

Depressed mood
Insomnia
Irritability, frustration, or anger
Anxiety
Difficulty concentrating
Restlessness
Decreased heart rate
Increased appetite or weight gain

How will you cope? Write your strategy for today here: _____. See Chapter 6 for a list of suggested coping strategies for withdrawal symptoms.

WHO'S STILL SMOKING?*

Smoking and Alcohol:

- Studies show that those who abuse alcohol are much more likely to smoke.
- In the general population, an estimated 20.8 percent of all adults (45.3 million people) smoke cigarettes in the United States.
- But among those who abuse or are dependent upon alcohol, an astonishing 56.1 percent are current smokers and 67.5 percent have smoked at some time in their lives.

* K. Lasser et al., "Smoking and Mental Illness: A Population-Based Prevalence Study," *JAMA*, 284, 20 (November 22–29, 2000).

BREAKING THE CONNECTION BETWEEN SMOKING AND DRINKING

At 6 weeks smoke-free and 3½ months sober, William M. got upset, angry, and disappointed and smoked two cigarettes. He was realizing that "being perfect" was not a healthy expectation! Over the next few months he began to recognize and admit to himself different "negative and anxious" feelings, which normally would have been covered over by drinking and smoking. He went on and off tobacco a number of times, usually in response to a wave, or a "flood," of anxiety. He began to learn to work with his emotional ups and downs, sadness, emptiness, frustration, bad moods, or just feeling blah. Life was far from the perfect vision he had imagined it would be when he got sober and quit smoking, but he was enjoying it more, and he was starting to like himself better.

DAY 19

Look at your calendar this evening to anticipate problems and develop strategies for tomorrow. For example, will there be stress, another smoker, or a gathering with smoking or alcohol, and how do you plan to handle these triggers?

Quote of the Day

"My taste buds are different and better. I've started walking half an hour a day. It helps with the frustrated energy or anxiety."

STRATEGY OF THE DAY

Walking has been shown to help with weight loss, cardio-vascular strength, muscular endurance, and bone strength. It is also a safe, enjoyable, and accessible way to get some exercise, and burn off some stress. We highly recommend it!

TASKS FOR THE DAY

Triggers to Watch Out For Today
Other smokers, alcohol, stress, other triggers.

Chart Your Cravings Today
Low, medium, high.

Chart Your Mood Today
Good, fair, upset, very upset.

Journal
Write in your journal how you plan in advance to handle today's triggers, and how you will cope with your cravings and mood today and tomorrow without smoking!

COPING WITH NICOTINE WITHDRAWAL SYMPTOMS IF YOU HAVE THEM

Note which symptoms you have today.

Depressed mood
Insomnia
Irritability, frustration, or anger
Anxiety
Difficulty concentrating
Restlessness

Decreased heart rate

Increased appetite or weight gain

How will you cope? Write your strategy for today in your journal. See Chapter 6 for a list of suggested coping strategies for withdrawal symptoms.

WHEN THE TRIGGER IS OTHER SMOKERS

Some people find that it helps not to linger around smokers; acknowledge the smoking person and move quickly to a nonsmoking place and interact with nonsmokers. People usually will try to help, so let them know you are no longer smoking. If you want, blame me and this book; just say that a doctor told you to avoid other smokers until a time when you won't be tempted. Meet smoking friends in nonsmoking environments, or put off seeing them for a while until you are on solid ground as a nonsmoker.

WHEN SMOKERS IN YOUR LIFE CAN'T OR WON'T BE SUPPORTIVE

In my experience, there is a lot of goodwill out there for someone trying to quit. Most friends and loved ones will want to help and will be supportive of your efforts, especially if you make specific requests of them. However, it isn't always this way. Sometimes it can be difficult to get family support. If you're in this situation, reread the section on being assertive with smokers in your life (pages 143–44).

DAY 20

Look at your calendar this evening to anticipate problems and develop strategies for tomorrow. For example, will there be stress, another smoker, or a gathering with smoking or alcohol, and how do you plan to handle these triggers?

Quote of the Day

> *"In my dream I smoked, and I felt it was because I was around smokers during the day. I made the connection between being with smokers and smoking."*

HONING YOUR MENTAL ATTITUDE

Dreams of smoking are not at all rare. They usually involve some element of bad conscience. "I smoked and felt bad about it." They are often so vivid that the person wakes up and is worried that the smoking really happened! Don't worry—dreams of smoking don't predict you will smoke in your real life when you are awake.

TASKS FOR THE DAY

Triggers to Watch Out For Today
Other smokers, alcohol, stress, other triggers.

Chart Your Cravings Today
Low, medium, high.

Chart Your Mood Today
Good, fair, upset, very upset.

Journal
Write in your journal how you plan in advance to handle today's triggers, and how you will cope with your cravings and mood today and tomorrow without smoking.

Good luck today and have a good day!

COPING WITH NICOTINE WITHDRAWAL SYMPTOMS IF YOU HAVE THEM

Note which symptoms you have today.

Depressed mood

Insomnia

Irritability, frustration, or anger

Anxiety

Difficulty concentrating

Restlessness

Decreased heart rate

Increased appetite or weight gain

How will you cope? Write your strategy for today in your journal. See Chapter 6 for a list of suggested coping strategies for withdrawal symptoms.

MINDFUL EATING

In my discussions with my colleague Dr. Erin Olivo, an authority on the mind-body connection, she emphasized that it is possible to cultivate mindfulness and increase our ability to be "awake" and "aware" during every activity we engage in. Eating is one activity that can definitely benefit from mindful attention. As Dr. Olivo explains it, all too often we eat unmindfully, perhaps not even tasting or fully experiencing our food, or even noticing how much we are eating! When we eat unmindfully, we aren't paying attention to the choices we are making and how they could ultimately be ineffective in our attempt to reach our health goals. With practice, mindful eating allows for the possibility that you can free yourself from habitual patterns of thinking, feeling, and acting on urges that are not healthy or effective. Mindfulness promotes balance, wisdom, and more effective choices. A person who eats mindfully has a greater awareness of the physical cues of hunger and satiety, a greater awareness of the full sensory experience of eating, and a greater insight about how food choices fit in with health goals.

Try this simple "mindful eating" exercise the next time you eat:*

- As you prepare to eat, take a moment to become aware of your body and your hunger or urge to eat.
- As you take your first bite, slow down and become aware of your movements as you bring the food to your mouth.
- Once the food is in your mouth, put down anything you have in your hands, such as your fork or any other food.
- As you chew this bite, bring awareness to just this moment of chewing. Bring your full concentration to the taste of the food, the texture of the food, and the sensation of eating. Don't do anything else while you are eating this bite. Simply chew and pay attention.
- When you are ready to swallow, take a moment to form an intention in your mind to swallow before doing so.
- After you swallow, take a moment to notice the sensation before picking up your fork or food for your next bite.
- Repeat this slow, deliberate way of eating with attention and awareness, pausing for a moment between each bite.

* From Erin Olivo, Ph.D., MPH, Columbia University Medical Center; used with permission.

DAY 21

Look at your calendar this evening to anticipate problems and develop strategies for tomorrow. For example, will there be stress, another smoker, or a gathering with smoking or alcohol, and how do you plan to handle these triggers

Quote of the Day

> *"Sometimes the craving is there. I just try to distract myself. I've learned it will be for just a few minutes. My wife is dealing with stronger cravings and is still using the nicotine inhaler when she gets them."*

STRATEGY OF THE DAY

The Greeks said, "Know thyself." The key to coping successfully with smoking is knowing what you need, which is different for different people and at different times as you adjust to no longer smoking.

TASKS FOR THE DAY

Triggers to Watch Out For Today
Other smokers, alcohol, stress, other triggers.

Chart Your Cravings Today
Low, medium, high.

Chart Your Mood Today
Good, fair, upset, very upset.

Journal

Write in your journal how you plan in advance to handle today's triggers, and how you will cope with your cravings and mood today and tomorrow without smoking.

COPING WITH NICOTINE WITHDRAWAL SYMPTOMS IF YOU HAVE THEM

Note which symptoms you have today.

Depressed mood

Insomnia

Irritability, frustration, or anger

Anxiety

Difficulty concentrating

Restlessness

Decreased heart rate

Increased appetite or weight gain

How will you cope? Write your strategy for today in your journal. See Chapter 6 for a list of suggested coping strategies for withdrawal symptoms.

DAY 22

Look at your calendar this evening to anticipate problems and develop strategies for tomorrow. For example, will there be stress, another smoker, or a gathering with smoking or alcohol, and how do you plan to handle these triggers? Also, chart your progress, including the ups and downs of cravings and moods, in the first 3 weeks of quitting for good!

HEALTH BENEFITS OF QUITTING*

Compared with the risk incurred by smokers, your . . .

- Risk of **stroke** is reduced to that of a person who never smoked after 5 to 15 years of not smoking.
- Risk of **cancers of the mouth, throat, and esophagus** are cut in half by 5 years after quitting.
- Risk of **cancer of the larynx** is reduced after quitting.
- Risk of **coronary heart disease** is cut by half 1 year after quitting and is nearly the same as that of someone who never smoked by 15 years after quitting.
- Risk of death from **chronic obstructive pulmonary disease** is reduced after you quit.
- Risk of **lung cancer** drops by as much as half 10 years after quitting.
- Risk of **ulcer** drops after quitting.
- Risk of **bladder cancer** is halved a few years after quitting.
- Risk of **peripheral artery disease** goes down after quitting.
- Risk of **cervical cancer** is reduced a few years after quitting.
- Risk of a **low-birth-weight baby** drops to normal if you quit before pregnancy or during your first trimester.

* Surgeon General's Report, *The Health Consequences of Smoking* (2004).

Quote of the Day

"I'm sleepy in the morning and used cigarettes and coffee to wake myself up. The rest of the day I didn't drink coffee or smoke. Coffee and smoking go together. I smell the coffee when making it, and it makes me automatically think of smoking. I will try regular tea instead and then switch to decaf tea."

STRATEGY OF THE DAY

Develop a new wake-up ritual. The smell of the coffee triggers a powerful response to smoke. Try not to test yourself, especially at first. It's easier for some people to avoid certain triggers, like coffee; or to limit their exposure to triggers, as with alcohol.

TASKS FOR THE DAY

Triggers to Watch Out For Today
Other smokers, alcohol, stress, other triggers.

Chart Your Cravings Today
Low, medium, high.

Chart Your Mood Today
Good, fair, upset, very upset.

Journal
Write in your journal how you plan in advance to handle today's triggers, and how you will cope with your cravings and mood today and tomorrow without smoking.

COPING WITH NICOTINE WITHDRAWAL SYMPTOMS IF YOU HAVE THEM

Note which symptoms you have today.

    Depressed mood
    Insomnia
    Irritability, frustration, or anger

Anxiety

Difficulty concentrating

Restlessness

Decreased heart rate

Increased appetite or weight gain

How will you cope? Write your strategy for today in your journal. See Chapter 6 for a list of suggested coping strategies for withdrawal symptoms.

BREATHING EASIER FOR LIFE

One day a man with emphysema arrived at our clinic pale as a ghost, seemingly at death's door. He was on a waiting list for a lung transplant, and needed to carry a tank of oxygen just to get to the appointment. I had always heard that emphysema patients who quit smoking don't get better; they just don't get worse, except for an age-related decline in their lung function This man, however, soon began to look more alive after going smoke-free. Eventually, he started showing up at the clinic without his oxygen tank!

More than a year after stopping smoking, he said he never used his oxygen anymore. If this kind of improvement is possible in someone with advanced emphysema, imagine how much more easily you will be able to breathe, and the health benefits you will enjoy, not just today, but every day for the rest of your life.

DAY 23

Look at your calendar this evening to anticipate problems and develop strategies for tomorrow. For example, will there be stress, another smoker, or a gathering with smoking or alcohol, and how do you plan to handle these triggers?

Quote of the Day

> *"The cravings are there—but I'm not close to smoking, because I know how to manage that craving."*

STRATEGY OF THE DAY

"I ask visitors to smoke out the window. If I really feel like smoking, I throw them out of the apartment. No matter what, even if someone dies, I will not smoke. I just have to learn how to deal with that problem."

TASKS FOR THE DAY

Triggers to Watch Out For Today
Other smokers, alcohol, stress, other triggers.

Chart Your Cravings Today
Low, medium, high.

Chart Your Mood Today
Good, fair, upset, very upset.

Journal
Write in your journal how you plan in advance to handle today's triggers, and how you will cope with your cravings and mood today and tomorrow without smoking.

COPING WITH NICOTINE WITHDRAWAL SYMPTOMS IF YOU HAVE THEM

Note which symptoms you have today.

Depressed mood
Insomnia

Irritability, frustration, or anger
Anxiety
Difficulty concentrating
Restlessness
Decreased heart rate
Increased appetite or weight gain

How will you cope? Write your strategy for today in your journal. See Chapter 6 for a list of suggested coping strategies for withdrawal symptoms.

WHAT I WOULD TELL YOU IF I COULD SIT DOWN WITH YOU IN PERSON . . .

"I haven't smoked for 2 weeks! The first week was less hard, the second week more difficult. The cigarette is telling me to smoke so I will be in control, but it doesn't put me in control; it puts me out of control. It's definitely a mind game! It's not really when I'm upset but when I'm short-circuited that I want it. The addiction says, 'Take a break; sit back and take a cigarette.' I've been taking tea when I need a break instead. The thing I'm enjoying the most is outsmarting the addiction! I'm using the 14-mg patch every day and about 1 cartridge of the inhaler a day, which is just something to do. I drink water, and I breathe deeply—this is particularly good for me. My friend is still smoking, and I sometimes see his cigarettes, which bother me and make me think I should have just one."

We often see a battle for control—a civil war within the smoker. On the one hand, smokers have a powerful wish to control the addiction (by smoking in a controlled manner). On the other hand, they may feel guilty about, or ashamed of, the addiction and embarrassed to be doing something so harmful to their health. There's usually an emotional disconnect between these different parts of the person. The job is to break down the wall separating the two sides so the person can become and feel whole again. Only when you repair that disconnect, and give up that battle to control, can you find peace.

Picture the ancient reptilian part of your brain versus the more modern, smart part of your brain. The old brain just wants what it wants when it wants it. It doesn't care about your body or even about reality! The smart brain is the educated, cultured part, which is *rational* and *realistic*. It is important to build up the smart brain so it can consolidate control, like a new government when it takes the reins of power. The addiction may seem to go away, but lives on as a kind of opposition party, organizing in the wilderness, hoping and waiting patiently for its return to power. It will exploit any weakness to return to the body politic. Just as an opportunistic infection seizes on a weakened immune system, smoking addiction seizes on the smoker's attempt to try "just one."

DAY 24

Look at your appointment calendar this evening to anticipate problems and develop strategies for tomorrow. For example, will there be stress, another smoker, or a gathering with smoking or alcohol, and how do you plan to handle these triggers?

Quote of the Day

> *"I have been dreaming about smoking. I was feeling guilty because in my last dream I was smoking a cigarette. It was Saturday night, and I was out drinking with friends. When I saw the others cigarettes, that was a dangerous moment for me, not only in the dream but in real life. In the dream I said, 'I can't fool myself; let me just stop and go speak to my nonsmoking buddy.' "*

STRATEGY OF THE DAY

Excuses to smoke can be dangerous. Getting better and being honest about what is an excuse go hand in hand.

TASKS FOR THE DAY

Triggers to Watch Out For Today
Other smokers, alcohol, stress, other triggers.

Chart Your Cravings Today
Low, medium, high.

Chart Your Mood Today
Good, fair, upset, very upset.

Journal
Write in your journal how you plan in advance to handle today's triggers, and how you will cope with your cravings and mood today and tomorrow without smoking.

COPING WITH NICOTINE WITHDRAWAL SYMPTOMS IF YOU HAVE THEM

Note which withdrawal symptoms apply to you today.

Depressed mood

Insomnia

Irritability, frustration, or anger

Anxiety

Difficulty concentrating

Restlessness

Decreased heart rate

Increased appetite or weight gain

IMMEDIATE REWARDS OF QUITTING*

Kicking the tobacco habit offers some benefits that you'll notice right away and some that will develop over time. These rewards can improve your day-to-day life a great deal.

Your breath smells better.

Stained teeth get whiter.

The bad smell goes away from your clothes and hair.

The yellow in your fingers and fingernails disappears.

Food tastes better.

Your sense of smell returns to normal.

Everyday activities (for example, climbing stairs and doing light housework) no longer leave you out of breath.

* American Cancer Society (2008).

How will you cope? Write your strategy for today in your journal. See Chapter 6 for a list of suggested coping strategies for withdrawal symptoms.

DAY 25

Look at your appointment calendar this evening to anticipate problems and develop strategies for tomorrow. For example, will there be stress, another smoker, or a gathering with smoking or alcohol, and how do you plan to handle these triggers? Also continue charting your progress, including the ups and downs of cravings and moods.

Quote of the Day

"It's been 2 weeks and 2 days. At first it was minute to minute, now it might happen only three times a day. Sometimes I even forget about it."

STRATEGY OF THE DAY

Learn what to do when cravings arise. One person says, "I distract myself by singing, exercising, or reading a book. I call someone on the phone; at the end of the call the craving is over."

TASKS FOR THE DAY

Triggers to Watch Out For Today
Other smokers, alcohol, stress, other triggers.

Chart Your Cravings Today
Low, medium, high.

Chart Your Mood Today
Good, fair, upset, very upset.

Journal
Write in your journal how you plan in advance to handle today's triggers, and how you will cope with your cravings and mood today and tomorrow without smoking.

COPING WITH NICOTINE WITHDRAWAL SYMPTOMS IF YOU HAVE THEM

Note which withdrawal symptoms apply to you today.

Depressed mood
Insomnia
Irritability, frustration, or anger
Anxiety
Difficulty concentrating
Restlessness
Decreased heart rate
Increased appetite or weight gain

How will you cope? Write your strategy for today in your journal. See Chapter 6 for a list of suggested coping strategies for withdrawal symptoms.

20 MINUTES TO 15 YEARS: MEDICAL BENEFITS AFTER QUITTING*

- 20 minutes after quitting: your heart rate and blood pressure drop.
  A. Mahmud and J. Feely, "Effect of Smoking on Arterial Stiffness and Pulse Pressure Amplification," *Hypertension*, 41 (2003): 183.

- 12 hours after quitting: the carbon monoxide level in your blood drops to normal.
  U.S. Surgeon General's Report (1988), p. 202.
- 2 weeks to 3 months after quitting: your circulation improves and your lung function increases.
  U.S. Surgeon General's Report (1990), pp.193, 194, 196, 285, 323.
- 1 to 9 months after quitting: coughing and shortness of breath decrease; cilia (tiny hairlike structures that move mucus out of the lungs) regain normal function in the lungs, increasing the ability to handle mucus, clean the lungs, and reduce the risk of infection.
  U.S. Surgeon General's Report (1990), pp. 285–287, 304.
- 1 year after quitting: the excess risk of coronary heart disease is half that of a smoker.
  U.S. Surgeon General's Report (1990), p. vi.
- 5 years after quitting: your stroke risk is reduced to that of a nonsmoker 5 to 15 years after quitting.
  U.S. Surgeon General's Report (1990), p. vi.
- 10 years after quitting: the death rate from lung cancer is about half that of a continuing smoker. The risk of cancer of the mouth, throat, esophagus, bladder, cervix, and pancreas decreases.
  U.S. Surgeon General's Report (1990), pp. vi, 131, 148, 152, 155, 164, 166.
- 15 years after quitting: the risk of coronary heart disease is that of a nonsmoker.
  U.S. Surgeon General's Report (1990), p. vi.

* American Cancer Society (2008).

DAY 26

Look at your appointment calendar this evening to anticipate problems and develop strategies for tomorrow. For example, will there be stress, another smoker, or a gathering with smoking or alcohol, and how do you plan to handle these triggers?

Quote of the Day

> *"My cravings increase if I drink coffee, so I stopped. It's the best way to stay away from cigarettes. I'm not even feeling the cravings when I'm around smokers, although I'm avoiding them. My mood was always good, but it's even better now!"*

STRATEGY OF THE DAY

The Greeks said, "Know thyself." For this program, "Know thy triggers!" The clearer you are about your triggers, the more you will be able to protect yourself from a relapse.

TASKS FOR THE DAY

Triggers to Watch Out for Today
Other smokers, alcohol, stress, other triggers.

Chart your Cravings Today
Low, medium, high.

Chart Your Mood Today
Good, fair, upset, very upset.

Journal

Write in your journal how you plan in advance to handle today's triggers, and how you will cope with your cravings and mood today and tomorrow without smoking.

COPING WITH NICOTINE WITHDRAWAL SYMPTOMS IF YOU HAVE THEM

Note which withdrawal symptoms apply to you today.

Depressed mood

Insomnia

Irritability, frustration, or anger

Anxiety

Difficulty concentrating

Restlessness

Decreased heart rate

Increased appetite or weight gain

How will you cope? Write your strategy for today in your journal. See Chapter 6 for a list of suggested coping strategies for withdrawal symptoms.

A CASE STUDY FROM THE HISTORY BOOKS
Dr. F. was the first doctor to describe nicotine withdrawal syndrome. What if he had had NRT available to treat it?

Dr. F. was a smoker who became seriously ill and was able to stop, but subsequently relapsed back to smoking.

He was a physician with a long, distinguished career, but he continued to smoke despite multiple medical complications. He received repeated advice to stop smoking, due to a heart arrhythmia at age 38, and he once had abstained for 14 months, after briefly cutting down to a weekly cigar (from his usual 20 a day). He found not smoking a torture, though, and insisted that he needed cigars for his work.[1] In his early sixties, he continued to feel this way, calling his cigars "the stuff of work."[2]

By age 61, though, he noticed a painful swelling in his mouth, and by the time he was 67 the growths on his jaw and palate associated with heavy smoking could not be ignored. Alarmed, he consulted with his colleagues, including those attending to him medically. They all avoided using the word cancer, *although he had himself correctly guessed this as the nature of his condition. Who was this medically ill smoker who couldn't quit? None other than Sigmund Freud.*

Surgery was unavoidable, but it almost cost him his life. Freud underwent 30 or more minor—and some major— operations, to remove precancerous growths. Incredibly, he continued to aggravate them by smoking! A huge prosthesis had to be inserted in his oral and nasal cavity, which also required repeated painful readjustments during this period.[3]

Despite all this, he was still smoking and undergoing painful operations until 7 years later, when, at the age of 74, he developed a complete intolerance for cigars. At this time he wrote to a close friend: "I have completely given up smoking, after it had served me for precisely fifty years as protection and weapon in the combat with life. So I am better than before, but not happier."[4]

Sigmund Freud stopped smoking under duress but never made a positive emotional adjustment to his new state. He was an emotionally dependent smoker who never made peace with his addiction. He rationalized his smoking, despite the great pain and harm it had done him, until the last years of his life. What a powerful rationalization he pro-

vided: after all, who can question a man's need to work and provide for his family?

But what if he had quit permanently at 38? What if nicotine replacement had been available to ease his withdrawal and facilitate a happier long-term adjustment? Perhaps he would have suffered less and found enough emotional confidence to handle life's battles without smoking. Many men and women believe, like Freud, that they will not be as effective in their work life without smoking; they believe that they will no longer be promoted or that they will lose their edge. I have treated many successful people who explained their smoking as necessary for their work. They believe that smoking helps them concentrate and that they will lose their cognitive ability when they stop.

In all these cases, however, each person who used nicotine replacement therapy appropriately was able to resume a productive work life after he or she stopped smoking. Nicotine replacement can help make this transition much less difficult. But the higher hurdle was challenging the false-belief system—built on the chemical and emotional dependency to tobacco—that these people needed to smoke in order to work. When they stop to think about it, most people realize that smoking can't make them any more talented or smarter, and that not smoking therefore can't take these gifts away. Ultimately, to make peace, the smoker must challenge the belief that smoking tobacco is the "stuff of work" and necessary for the "combat with life"; the smoker must disconnect smoking from work.[5]

Like Sigmund Freud, many people who stop smoking never break their emotional dependency on it, and therefore are at high risk of a relapse. It is like the difference between pining away for an old lover and waiting for a chance to get back together, versus accepting that the person just wasn't for you, accepting the painful disappointment, and realizing that your life is now actually better.

NOTES

1. Ernest Jones, *The Life and Work of Sigmund Freud*, edited and abridged in 1 vol. by Lionel Trilling and Steven Marcus (New York: Basic Books, 1961), p. 202.

2. Peter Gay, *Freud: A Life for Our Time* (New York: Norton, 1988), p. 384.

3. Ibid., pp. 418–427.

4. Ibid., 573.

5. A review similar to this case study can be found in Sheldon Cohen, "Tobacco Addiction as a Psychiatric Disease" *Southern Medical Journal*, 81, 9 (September 1988): 1083–1088.

DAY 27

Look at your calendar this evening to anticipate problems and develop strategies for tomorrow. For example, will there be stress, another smoker, or a gathering with smoking or alcohol, and how do you plan to handle these triggers? Also, continue charting your progress, including the ups and downs of cravings and moods.

Quote of the Day

> "Smoking was my way to hide from and disobey my mother and her demands while I was growing up. Now I think of it when I'm anxious and insecure and I lose perspective. I never did learn to trust myself enough to openly disagree with my mother and others in my life."

STRATEGY OF THE DAY

Assertiveness is a high art. It often requires thinking through what you want and how best to present it to the specific person you are addressing. See the section on assertiveness (page 143).

TASKS FOR THE DAY

Triggers to Watch Out For Today
Other smokers, alcohol, stress, other triggers.

Chart Your Cravings Today
Low, medium, high.

Chart Your Mood Today
Good, fair, upset, very upset.

Journal
Write in your journal how you plan in advance to handle today's triggers, and how you will cope with your cravings and mood today and tomorrow without smoking.

COPING WITH NICOTINE WITHDRAWAL SYMPTOMS IF YOU HAVE THEM

Note which withdrawal symptoms apply to you today.

Depressed mood
Insomnia
Irritability, frustration, or anger
Anxiety
Difficulty concentrating

Restlessness
Decreased heart rate
Increased appetite or weight gain

How will you cope? Write your strategy for today in your journal. See Chapter 6 for a list of suggested coping strategies for withdrawal symptoms.

WHAT I WOULD TELL YOU IF I COULD SIT DOWN WITH YOU IN PERSON . . .

"Every time I visit my relatives I go for the weekend. On day one I'm fine, even though they all smoke. But on day two I smoke with them, even if I haven't been smoking for months before I visit."

Some people and places prove to be too much of a trigger to smoke. If you have to be with these people in these places, make plans to confine your visit to smoke-free environments or to a briefer time period.

DAY 28

Look at your appointment calendar this evening to anticipate problems and develop strategies for tomorrow. For example, will there be stress, another smoker, or a gathering with smoking or alcohol, and how do you plan to handle these triggers? Also, continue charting your progress, including the ups and downs of cravings and moods.

Quote of the day (from Someone 8 Months Smoke-Free)

"I still feel the craving, but the good part is that it is less intense and occurs less often. Now it is sometimes once a day, not every day. It could be three or four times a week at most, but at least once a week. It doesn't last long—just a couple of minutes—and it's related to things I used to do when I smoked, like drinking coffee or sitting around after a meal. I can handle it. I am not close to smoking because of cravings."

STRATEGY OF THE DAY

Over a long period of time cravings become more like thoughts, rather than a physical experience. Just remember that we have all kinds of thoughts. Thoughts by themselves don't harm us. They can just come and go.

TASKS FOR THE DAY

Triggers to Watch Out For Today
Other smokers, alcohol, stress, other triggers.

Chart Your Cravings Today
Low, medium, high.

Chart Your Mood Today
Good, fair, upset, very upset.

Journal
Write in your journal how you plan in advance to handle today's triggers, and how you will cope with your cravings and mood today and tomorrow without smoking.

COPING WITH NICOTINE WITHDRAWAL SYMPTOMS IF YOU HAVE THEM

Note which withdrawal symptoms apply to you today.

Depressed mood
Insomnia
Irritability, frustration, or anger
Anxiety
Difficulty concentrating
Restlessness
Decreased heart rate
Increased appetite or weight gain

How will you cope? Write your strategy for today in your journal. See Chapter 6 for a list of suggested coping strategies for withdrawal symptoms.

ON HAVING "JUST ONE"

"I was out of town on business, already feeling like a 'bad boy,' like a kid away from my parents. I was sitting in a bar with a friend having a few drinks, and he lit up. I asked him for a puff, and now it's months later. I'm back home and have been hiding my 10 cigarettes a day from my wife like a child."

Beware of the voice in your head that says, "Have just one." If you could have just one you wouldn't be addicted to smoking. This is an example of the kind of tricky thinking that you can have even after a long time away from cigarettes.

DAY 29

Look at your appointment calendar this evening to anticipate problems and develop strategies for tomorrow. For example, will there be stress, another smoker, or a gathering with smoking or alcohol, and how do you plan to handle these triggers? Also, continue charting your progress, including the ups and downs of cravings and moods.

Quote of the Day

"I do not want to relapse again. It's very hard for me when I crave a cigarette, but I know that smoking will not be the solution."

STRATEGY OF THE DAY

"I am working on not connecting personal problems with the urge to smoke. Some family members are making life difficult, and I am craving a cigarette, but they are two separate problems. I am feeling happier each day without smoking."

TASKS FOR THE DAY

Triggers to Watch Out For Today
Other smokers, alcohol, stress, other triggers.

Chart Your Cravings Today
Low, medium, high.

Chart Your Mood Today
Good, fair, upset, very upset.

Journal

Write in your journal how you plan in advance to handle today's triggers, and how you will cope with your cravings and mood today and tomorrow without smoking.

COPING WITH NICOTINE WITHDRAWAL SYMPTOMS IF YOU HAVE THEM

Note which withdrawal symptoms apply to you today.

Depressed mood

Insomnia

Irritability, frustration, or anger

Anxiety

Difficulty concentrating

Restlessness

Decreased heart rate

Increased appetite or weight gain

How will you cope? Write your strategy for today in your journal. See Chapter 6 for a list of suggested coping strategies for withdrawal symptoms and "Three Views on Not Having 'Just One' " on the next page.

DAY 30

Look at your calendar this evening to anticipate problems and develop strategies for tomorrow. For example, will there be stress, another smoker, or a gathering with smoking or alcohol, and how do you plan to handle these triggers?

THREE VIEWS ON NOT HAVING "JUST ONE"

"I didn't know before, and I learned the hard way that if I take one puff from a cigarette, that will be trouble for me."

"I feel free from smoking. I'm using the inhaler, sometimes when I am not craving, but as a preventive. I see so many people in treatment for drug relapse. If they do a little they lose control. I won't go back because of family problems. You have to be positive and focus only on that. I tell people the cigarette thrives on negativity. You have to be more positive. I am really, really proud. My skin is better, I am sleeping better, I am smelling better, my friends are noticing and complimenting me. I am eating better. All these things go together!"

"Yesterday morning I had some cravings; my body was asking for a cigarette. I have to realize that I shouldn't try at least one. I discuss it with my wife, and we distract and support each other. She is still using the inhaler, but I no longer need it. I have to do something with coffee. When I drink more coffee than usual I have cravings, like those I had yesterday. I am considering cutting down on coffee. My wife suggests I change the flavor and not use sugar but a substitute to help."

Quote of the Day

"I have been doing better and forgot the patch today. But my cravings have been increasing the last few hours."

STRATEGY OF THE DAY

People often stop using NRT too soon, while they still need it. Just as not having enough confidence can be a problem, overconfidence also can make problems. It's important to know when you are truly confident and comfortable about not needing NRT. This is the time to stop NRT, and not before.

TASKS FOR THE DAY

Triggers to Watch Out For Today
Other smokers, alcohol, stress, other triggers.

Chart Your Cravings Today
Low, medium, high.

Chart Your Mood Today
Good, fair, upset, very upset.

Journal
Write in your journal how you plan in advance to handle today's triggers, and how you will cope with your cravings and mood today and tomorrow without smoking.

COPING WITH NICOTINE WITHDRAWAL SYMPTOMS IF YOU HAVE THEM

Note which withdrawal symptoms apply to you today.

Depressed mood
Insomnia
Irritability, frustration, or anger
Anxiety
Difficulty concentrating
Restlessness
Decreased heart rate
Increased appetite or weight gain

How will you cope? Write your strategy for today in your journal. See Chapter 6 for a list of suggested coping strategies for withdrawal symptoms.

WHAT I WOULD TELL YOU IF I COULD SIT DOWN WITH YOU IN PERSON . . .

"I can't tell you how many times over the years I told myself, 'Just have one,' only to then have another and get back into smoking. I now see this for what it is: an excuse that doesn't work."

Addiction is like a wound. Remember when you got a cut as a child and your mother said, "Don't pick at it." Well, when you take "just one" cigarette, it's like pulling off the bandage and opening up the wound all over again. When you do this, you interrupt the healing in the brain and the mind, and risk becoming re-addicted.

A FINAL WORD

You may be the kind of smoker who no longer thinks about smoking now that you have quit. You are one of the lucky ones! But you may be someone who does return to thoughts of smoking during times of great emotional stress, because it was such an important way you tried to cope with overwhelming feelings. If this describes you, please continue to use this book to keep yourself from slipping back. Keep it handy and refer to it often. I know how hard quitting can be for some smokers, but my experience helping many smokers quit has taught me that success is possible. I hope this book will see you through to a new smoke-free life.

ACKNOWLEDGMENTS

This book would not exist without the help and support I have received over the past 20 years from colleagues at the Columbia University Medical Center. When I got my first job at Columbia, after training there as a clinical psychologist, I was introduced to Jeff Rosecan and Henry Spitz, who had just written a textbook on cocaine abuse and were running a busy program for cocaine abusers. They asked me to join them in leading groups of cocaine, alcohol, and other substance abusers, despite my lack of experience in this area. Jeff was that rare clinician in psychiatry who really understood how to work with addictions. He quickly became not just a colleague, opening up a whole new field to me, but a great friend.

At this same time, I also began working with Alexander Glassman, who was starting a smoking cessation research unit at the New York State Psychiatric Institute; and with

Lirio Covey, who had come to Columbia from the American Health Foundation to do psychiatric research on tobacco use. Sandy and Lirio have been leaders in understanding how psychiatric disorders contribute to smoking dependence. Through my association with these outstanding scientists, I began to see similarities among smokers, cocaine abusers, alcoholics, and heroin abusers. They all had to learn how to solve life's problems, and how to cope with mood problems or distress without their drugs.

Fifteen years ago I joined the Columbia University Behavioral Medicine Program under the direction of Richard Sloan. This group of talented researchers and clinicians, including Ethan Gorenstein, Kenneth Gorfinkle, Catherine Monk, Erin Olivo, and Felice Tager has provided me with a supportive and intellectually stimulating environment in which to develop my ideas and my approach to helping smokers. Richard Sloan has been a leader of this group, consistently acting as a loyal friend and supporter to the whole staff, and always bringing people with common interests together. It was Richard who introduced me to Ed Katkin and Steve Goldband, who opened up one of the most exciting chapters in my work with smokers. Ed, Steve, and I began discussing using smoking as a model to test whether the Internet could be harnessed for behavior change. We spent the next 5 years planning, developing, and testing our online clinic. Recently we presented our findings from a large-scale national research trial sponsored by the American Cancer Society, which showed that our interactive online method helped smokers stay smoke-free for a year.

For the past 12 years I have had the privilege of running a Tobacco Cessation Clinic at the Columbia University College of Dental Medicine. We began the clinic under the leadership of Dean Allan Formicola, who regretted that there had been no help available to him when he quit smoking. He became an unfailing supporter of the clinic and later led a joint effort funded by the W. K. Kellogg Foundation and the American Legacy Foundation addressing smoking prevention and cessation. The national Community Voices project, as this effort was called, developed 13 sites nationwide aimed at helping individuals in low-income communities who were disproportionately affected by tobacco and by advertising for tobacco. This funding helped us develop our clinic and also fund dozens of community-based youth antitobacco projects in Washington Heights and Harlem.

I am also grateful to the current dean, Ira Lamster, for his ongoing support of the tobacco cessation initiatives at the College of Dental Medicine. Dean Lamster's help and support in promoting tobacco cessation is in the best tradition of disease prevention, clinical care, and research, which has a strong history at the Columbia University College of Dental Medicine. Without the generous and good-natured help of Ronnie Myers, Lynn Tepper, Jim Fine, and David Albert, I would not have been able to deliver the services and training opportunities to students and faculty members that the College of Dental Medicine offers. There is no question as well that without our outreach coordinator Martin Ovalles, who has become the model community health worker for delivering tobacco cessation services, we could not have helped so many medically and psychiatrically ill smokers become tobacco-free.

Recently, I collaborated with Mehmet C. Oz, M.D., of Columbia University, and Michael F. Roizen, M.D., of the Cleveland Clinic on an entire *Oprah Winfrey Show* about smokers. I was inspired by Mehmet and Michael's approach to public health education: presenting complex information in terms that can benefit the largest number of people. Great thanks to Mehmet and Mike as well as J. Lee Westmaas, Ph.D., of the American Cancer Society for their generous and helpful suggestions and comments. I also want to thank Marina Picciotto, the Charles B.G. Murphy Professor of Psychiatry, Pharmacology, and Neurobiology at Yale University School of Medicine, for her willingness to review the section of this book describing the neurobiology of smoking. Kathleen O'Connell, the Isabel Maitland Stewart Professor of Nursing Education at Teachers College, Columbia University, was kind enough to review and comment on an early version of this book. Jennifer Josephy helped pull together the final version of this book, and I am very grateful to her. I also would like to acknowledge an exhibit, "Not a Cough in a Carload—Images from the Tobacco Industry Campaign to Hide the Hazards of Smoking," Collection of Stanford University (tobacco.stanford.edu), created by Robert K. Jackler, M.D., Robert N. Proctor, Ph.D., Laurie M. Jackler, and Rachel Jackler.

Richard Pine, Susan Arellano, and Elisa Petrini have guided me as my agent-editors at Inkwell Management. Michelle Howry, my editor at Touchstone/Fireside Simon & Schuster, has been a patient, insightful, and enthusiastic editor. As always, my wife, Susan, has been generous with her editorial advice and expertise.

RESOURCES

Information from the American Cancer Society is available on the Web at: www.cancer.org. Click on Guide to Quitting Smoking. Telephone: 1-800-ACS-2345.

Other sources of information and support include:

American Heart Association and American
Stroke Association
Telephone: 1-800-AHA-USA-1 or 1-800-242-8721
Telephone: 1-888-4-STROKE or 1-888-478-7653
Internet address: www.amhrt.org
Internet address: www.strokeassociation.org

American Lung Association
Telephone: 1-800-LUNG-USA (1-800-548-8252)
Internet address: www.lungusa.org

Centers for Disease Control and Prevention
Office on Smoking and Health
Telephone: 1-800-CDC-INFO (1-800-232-4636)
Internet address: www.cdc.gov/tobacco

National Cancer Institute
Cancer Information Service
Telephone: 1-800-4-CANCER (1-800-422-6237)
Internet address: www.cancer.gov
Quitlines at 1-800-QUIT-NOW

National Institute on Drug Abuse
Internet address: www.nida.nih.gov

Nicotine Anonymous
Telephone: 1-877-879-6422
Internet address: www.nicotine-anonymous.org

Smokefree.gov
(Online materials, including information on state telephone-based programs)
Telephone: 1-877-44U-QUIT
Internet address: www.smokefree.gov

Smoking Cessation Leadership Center
Internet address: http://smokingcessationleadership.ucsf
.edu

INDEX

Abrams, David, 13
acupuncture, 162
addiction, 14, 47, 150
  alcoholism and, 33–36
  characteristics of, 129–30
  creative rationalization and, 27
  emotional dependency and,
    12–13, 30, 193–96
  Fagerström test for nicotine,
    116–17
  30-day schedule and, 120,
    129–30, 131, 166, 185–86, 205
Addiction, 77n
"addictive personalities," 36
advertising, 17–20, *18, 19,* 21, 22
aging, 15, 33, 133
alcohol, alcoholics, 27, 43
  case histories of, 33–35, 97, 101,
    173
  health questionnaire for, 74–75
  relapse and, 95, 103, 105–6
  30-day schedule and, 137, 143,
    146, 167, 172
American Cancer Society, 5, 67,
    125

American Journal of Public Health,
    25n
American Psychiatric Association,
    88, 118
anger, 29–30, 78
  case histories of, 27–28, 29–30,
    97–98, 101
  30-day schedule and, 127
  withdrawal and, 90–91, 101
Annals of Internal Medicine,
    33n
Antabuse, 34
anxiety, 30
  health questionnaire for, 72–73
  30-day schedule and, 119–20,
    156, 159, 196
  withdrawal and, 91
appetite increase, 92–93
assertiveness, 143–44, 197

behavioral changes, 2, 80–82, 115,
    137–38, 143
Bjartveit, K., 5
bladder cancer, 181, 191
Bogart, Humphrey, 19–20

ABOUT THE AUTHOR

DANIEL F. SEIDMAN, Ph.D., is a member of the Columbia University Behavioral Medicine Faculty, and a practicing psychotherapist. He is Assistant Clinical Professor of Medical Psychology at the Columbia University College of Physicians and Surgeons, and Director of Smoking Cessation Services at the Columbia University Behavioral Medicine Program. His practice includes adults and older adolescents, and he has extensive experience with addiction and psychotherapy.

DR. SEIDMAN is coeditor of and a contributing author to the book *Helping the Hard-Core Smoker: A Clinician's Guide* (1999). His research interests include developing innovative approaches to assist underserved and highly addicted smokers. He is also currently a consultant at the Naomi Berrie Diabetes Center at Columbia University Medical Center.

DR. SEIDMAN has made extensive appearances in the media, including *The Oprah Winfrey Show*, the XM radio show *Oprah and Friends* with Dr. Oz and BBC Radio. He has also been interviewed as an expert for articles in the *Wall Street Journal*, *New York* magazine, *BusinessWeek*, *AMNews (The Newspaper for America's Physicians)* and has made frequent appearances on local television programs and in other media. He has a Ph.D. in clinical psychology from Columbia University.